12 WAYS
TO AGE GRACEFULLY

HOW TO LOOK AND FEEL YOUNGER

SUSAN U. NEAL
RN, MBA, MHS

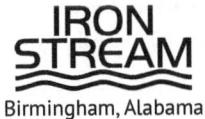

Birmingham, Alabama

12 Ways to Age Gracefully

Iron Stream
An imprint of Iron Stream Media
100 Missionary Ridge
Birmingham, AL 35242
IronStreamMedia.com

Copyright © 2024 by Susan U. Neal

Library of Congress Control Number: 2023950047

ISBN: 978-1-56309-686-0 (paperback)
ISBN: 978-1-56309-687-7 (eBook)

No part of this publication may be reproduced, stored in a retrieval system, or transmitted in any form or by any means—electronic, mechanical, photocopying, recording, or otherwise—without the prior written permission of the publisher.

Iron Stream Media serves its authors as they express their views, which may not express the views of the publisher. The information provided in this book does not constitute an endorsement by Iron Stream Media.

Unless otherwise indicated, all Scripture quotations are taken from the Holy Bible, New Living Translation, copyright © 1996, 2004, 2015 by Tyndale House Foundation. Used by permission of Tyndale House Publishers, Carol Stream, Illinois 60188. All rights reserved.

Scripture marked GW is taken from *GOD'S WORD*®. © 1995, 2003, 2013, 2014, 2019, 2020 by God's Word to the Nations Mission Society. Used by permission.

Scripture quotations marked (NIV) are taken from the Holy Bible, New International Version®, NIV®. Copyright © 1973, 1978, 1984, 2011 by Biblica, Inc.™ Used by permission of Zondervan. All rights reserved worldwide. www.zondervan.com The "NIV" and "New International Version" are trademarks registered in the United States Patent and Trademark Office by Biblica, Inc.™

Scripture quotations marked (TLB) are taken from The Living Bible, copyright © 1971 by Tyndale House Foundation. Used by permission of Tyndale House Publishers, Carol Stream, Illinois 60188. All rights reserved.

Cover design by twolineSTUDIO.com

1 2 3 4 5—28 27 26 25 24

"In *12 Ways to Age Gracefully*, Susan Neal weaves relatable stories from her personal health journey with her extensive dietary expertise resulting in an empowering guide that reads like a conversation with a trusted friend. From dietary insights to scriptural wisdom, Susan provides readers with actionable strategies to help them prioritize wellness in every area of their lives." **Dr. Saundra Dalton-Smith**, physician, best-selling author, and host of *I Choose My Best Life* podcast

"In *12 Ways to Age Gracefully*, Susan Neal shares from her own personal experience to help the reader understand the ways our mind, body, and spirit interact to affect our health and impact the aging process." **Dr. Michelle Bengtson**, author of *Breaking Anxiety's Grip*

"*12 Ways to Age Gracefully* is an empowering and transformative guide, revealing the secrets to rejuvenating your spirit and body, aligning perfectly with God's plan for a vibrant, purposeful life at any age—a must-read for those seeking to renew their zest for life!" **Laine Lawson Craft**, best-selling and award-winning author, *Warfare Parenting* podcast host, and speaker

"*12 Ways to Age Gracefully* explains how to make better decisions in diet and physical activities. The book provides well-balanced applications for issues we face as we age, including our spiritual health. Through this book, we learn the secrets to healthy habits and a long life." **Billie Jauss**, international speaker, author of *Making Room*, *Distraction Detox*, and *Baseball Family*, and host of *The Family Room* podcast

"Susan Neal shares how she overcame ten serious medical problems that impacted her lifespan. The information includes checklists of conditions related to various problems and changes to make in response. She covers health, emotional, mental, and physical choices for a better, longer life, to start at any age." **Karen Whiting**, award-winning author, coach, international speaker, and former television host

"Best-selling author Susan Neal has the perfect recipe for aging gracefully. Combining years of health services experience with the education and wisdom of her registered nurse occupation, Neal offers 12 tips, explained in detail with personal and practical applications, to help the reader find joy and meaning in growing older while growing closer to the Lord and maintaining healthy habits for a long life. This one's a keeper for any age!" **Julie Lavender**, author of *Strength for All Seasons* and *Children's Bible Stories for Bedtime*

"*12 Ways to Age Gracefully* stands as a must-read to optimize our quality of life as we mature. Readers will discover the scrumptious joys of living their best. This practical guide addresses every area of our lifestyle with specific steps to vitalize our golden years. I will recommend this book to my clients, and I look forward to gifting copies to loved ones." **Tina Yeager**, LMHC, life coach, *Flourish-Meant* podcast host, speaker, and award-winning author

"*12 Ways to Age Gracefully* is a comprehensive approach to addressing age-related health issues we often assume to be unavoidable. Eschewing anti-aging fads, Susan provides practical information to help regain health and wholeness. This book will be an invaluable resource that readers will refer to again and again!" **Ava Pennington**, MBA, speaker, Bible teacher, freelance editor, and author of *Reflections on the Names of God*

"Susan Neal is the perfect example of one who practices what she preaches. In this informative book, she covers every aspect of our lives and explains how to maintain a healthy balance in all of them. Presented in a well-organized, thorough manner, Neal provides interesting insight about how to maintain and achieve our health despite the normal results of getting older. This is a book you will want to read and keep on hand to refer to from time to time. I know I will!" **Marilyn Turk**, award-winning author of *The Escape Game*

"Whether you're already in your senior years or not there yet, the best time to begin aging gracefully is today. Susan shares her own poor health experiences, which motivate her ongoing journey to better health. As a nurse and certified health and wellness coach, she has the medical background and training to understand and explain groundbreaking research in ways everyday people can use in their lives. Whatever your dreams are for your senior years, you'll want to feel good and have the energy to enjoy them fully. Get started today. I have." **Ginny Cruz**, PT, MPA, author of *The New Mom's Guide*

"Susan Neal's excellent new book on aging gracefully is research-based and practical. She fought her own health crisis with ten diagnoses and two surgeries. Doctors could not heal her, so she has used her nursing and health science background to learn how to regain her health. The author of several books on healthy eating, she is now on a mission to help others like me look better and live longer. I can't recommend this enough!" **Janet Holm McHenry**, author of 26 books, including the best-selling *PrayerWalk*

"All throughout this book, I felt like Susan was talking directly to me! I could see myself in so many of the issues that plague people today. Through her extensive experience and expertise as a registered nurse and certified health coach, she provides encouragement for all of us struggling with the aging process that we can age not only gracefully but also victoriously." **Michelle S. Lazurek**, multi-genre award-winning author of *Who God Wants Me to Be*

"What impresses me most about Susan Neal's *12 Ways to Age Gracefully* is Susan's simple approach: do this, not that. And the bonus? She explains *why*. For someone like me who isn't versed in medical terminology, Susan's book is a refreshing resource I find easy to understand and will use as a reference for the rest of my life. I already have a list of questions to review with my doctor during my next visit. Thanks, Susan!" **Shellie Arnold**, author, speaker, and biblical marriage strategist

"My desire as I age is to finish well. Susan gives you practical tips for aging with grace and good health while leaving a legacy of faith. A *must-read* for all who desire to finish well!" **Ginny Dent Brant**, speaker and author of *Unleash Your God-Given Healing*

"The author presents well-researched, extensive guidelines on the day-to-day impact of choices we can make in life. *12 Ways to Age Gracefully* motivates the reader to contemplate the given advice and motivates them to make changes that are realistic. The "12 Ways" edify and encourage with simplicity and applicability for all to embrace. This book is for those who wish to live a healthy, vibrant, fully functional life, walking out their God-given path." **Rick Bennett**, MD

"This is an excellent comprehensive book that details the various vital areas of health and how it can positively impact longevity. A healthy body and mind that work together are absolutely essential. The author has done a great job emphasizing both the biochemical and psychological components that contribute to overall well-being. Most importantly, you will get a healthy dose of scripture along with it." **Adam Cabaniss**, DC

"*12 Ways to Age Gracefully* by Susan Neal offers a commonsense, no nonsense, holistic approach to aging. The approachable, organized structure invites the reader to choose actionable, attainable goals. While reading, I was repeatedly reminded of the exhortation of Jesus—physician, heal thyself! In response, I have chosen to apply one goal each month for the next year and look forward to the positive transformation." **Linda J. Dindzans**, MD, author of *A Certain Man*

"Whether you are just starting your wellness journey or on the path to longevity, *12 Ways to Age Gracefully* is the ultimate resource to guide you every step of the way. You can reclaim that youthful energy and glow and keep disease and illness from claiming you as its next victim. Susan offers practical advice in addition to the best proven scientific methods. You will want to reference this book often and give it to the ones you love!" **Lee Ann Mancini**, author of *Raising Kids to Follow Christ*, podcast host of *Raising Christian Kids*

"Another self-help book? Most urge a strict path that is all too often unsustainable. This book does it a bit differently. A gem is that she reinforces a time-honored strategy that we too often abandon: the therapeutic trial. If you think you have an issue and you pursue it with a supplement, treatment, or avoidance and nothing changes, try a different path. She lists numerous courses of actions to test with many how-to suggestions. Most importantly, this book emphasizes to "take care of the temple God gave you." We are made in his image, his greatest gift, and none wish to be found wanting in caring for that gift. Read this book." **Dennis Mayeaux**, MD

"Susan Neal has beautifully captured the keys to living life up to our God-given potential in her book *12 Ways to Age Gracefully*. Susan covers all the bases. She has literally unlocked the doors we all seek to walk through in achieving our most fulfilling life, the one God has designed for us. This book is a must-read; it is changing my life—it will change yours too." **John Rabins**, PhD, OD, author of *Defined by Fire*

I dedicate this book to my mother-in-law, Sue Neal, who inspired me to broaden my medical-driven perspective to a holistic approach to prevent disease, live longer, and stay healthy your entire life.

DISCLAIMER: Although I am a nurse and health care professional, I am not your personal health care professional. All content and information in this book is for informational and educational purposes only, does not constitute medical advice, and does not establish any kind of patient-client relationship by your reading of this book. People concerned about their diet or health should seek the advice of a licensed medical doctor. The information in this book is intended as a guide only and not representative of medical advice. Always seek the advice of your physician or other qualified health care provider with any questions you may have regarding a medical condition or treatment and before undertaking a new health care regimen, and never disregard professional medical advice or delay in seeking it because of something you read in this book.

CONTENTS

Introduction xi

Chapter 1: Eat to Live Longer 1

Chapter 2: Keep Your Gut Healthy 22

Chapter 3: The Secret to Staying Physically Active 38

Chapter 4: Keep Your Brain Young 58

Chapter 5: Eliminate Toxins: Inside and Out 70

Chapter 6: Balance and Stabilize Your Hormones 86

Chapter 7: Overcome the Battle with Stress 102

Chapter 8: Maintain a Positive Emotional Life 119

Chapter 9: Guard Your Mental Health 133

Chapter 10: Created for Work, Community, and Balance 146

Chapter 11: Cultivate Your Spiritual Health 163

Chapter 12: Healthy Habits for a Long Life 175

Appendix: Fall Prevention 187

Notes 189

INTRODUCTION

There is one consolation in being sick; and that is the possibility that you may recover to a better state than you were ever in before.
—Henry David Thoreau

Imagine you wake up the morning of your seventy-fifth or eightieth birthday and struggle to get out of bed. You are unable to play with your grandchildren when they come to celebrate this milestone day with you. You have no energy to enjoy your family and friends. The thought of another new day of life is exhausting. You're too tired to dream about anything better.

Now, imagine yourself on that same birthday, eagerly arising to greet the morning and commemorate this occasion. You're fit and able to prepare your home, cook a meal, and greet your family when they arrive. You have the energy to enjoy your grandchildren and laugh and reminisce with all your friends and family. You rest your head that evening with a satisfied smile and look forward to the next day. You dream about the next trip you plan to take. You are proud of the way you look and feel.

Which version of your future self would you prefer? Obviously, we'd all choose the second scenario. You may have taken the steps to a healthier future already or have made choices in the past that lead down the other path. No matter where you are at this point in your life, you can apply the healthy living tips from this book to improve your health. On your next birthday, you'll look and feel younger than you do today by learning how to age gracefully.

Thank you for joining me on this journey to slow the aging process. While we can't go back in time—and our bodies will inevitably age—

we can maintain energy and even improve our health as we face each new day and live well into our golden years. I know. I learned this lesson the hard way.

MY HEALTH CRISIS

You could call me a health nut. I am a registered nurse with a master's degree in health science and a certified Christian health and wellness coach. I research and study healthy lifestyles, and I diligently seek to live one myself. My motto is "inspiring others to improve their health so they can serve God better." However, I wasn't always in such good shape.

I started this journey to help others recover their optimal health and weight and reverse the aging process after I suffered a health crisis at forty-nine. My problems started with a crown placed on my tooth. Over the next nine months, this tooth abscessed and poisoned my body, resulting in ten medical diagnoses and two surgeries. Yet this cause of all my health problems didn't come to light right away.

At first, I suffered from depression. A month after receiving the dental crown, I experienced two menstrual cycles per month. The double periods continued for fifteen months until I had surgery to remove two uterine polyps.

Next, my gynecologist diagnosed an ovarian cyst and a hormonal imbalance and prescribed progesterone cream for both. Two months later, I was diagnosed with adrenal fatigue, and my doctor recommended three different adrenal vitamins five times a day. With no stamina, I felt completely depleted.

A couple of months later, I suddenly saw flashes of light in my left eye when I quickly turned my head to the left. I had a hole in my retina. The ophthalmologist performed emergency surgery since retinal tears can lead to blindness if the retina becomes detached. Even today, when I turn my head sharply to the left, I still see a flash of light. I will never regain that part of my vision.

Soon after eye surgery, I began to experience visual migraines even though I had never suffered from headaches. That month I went to my dentist for a cleaning, and finally he discovered the previously crowned tooth was abscessed. I had an emergency root canal along with ten days of antibiotics and two weeks of steroids.

Afterward, I was so fatigued I could not put away the groceries after shopping. No one understood how depleted my system was because on the outside I looked fine. On the inside, however, I was a train wreck. My relationships with my husband and three children were frazzled. They didn't understand why I couldn't keep up with the housework, grocery shopping, and cooking. Everything in our home and my life was a mess.

My weight continued to increase as did my illness. At only fifty years of age, I had lost my health. All my life I had taken my good health for granted. Now, I realized it was precious and was not guaranteed.

On my fiftieth birthday, a friend gave me a plaque with this verse:

> Those who hope in the LORD
> will renew their strength.
> They will soar on wings like eagles;
> they will run and not grow weary,
> they will walk and not be faint.
> —Isaiah 40:31 NIV

At this point in my illness, I wondered if I might be better off dead. Still, I clung to this verse and hoped one day I would be well again.

Next, my doctor found I was anemic and low in vitamin D, so I took iron and vitamin D supplements. I felt utterly drained and could have easily stayed in bed every day, and this caused more strain and conflict with my family. My husband was upset that he and our daughters had to pick up the load in caring for our home and family because I never had the energy to do so.

When my medical doctors had done all they could for me, I sought alternative health care therapies, such as massage, acupuncture, and colonic irrigation (royal enema). The therapist found candida in my colon. Despite being a nurse, I had never heard of this type of infection because mainstream medicine did not teach about candidiasis of the gut (candida infection from a *Candida* fungus, a type of yeast) at that time. Even my internal medicine doctor didn't know how to rid me of this yeast infection.

People are more prone to getting yeast infections when they take antibiotics because these drugs kill off beneficial flora in the body. I had just consumed antibiotics and a steroid, which killed the probiotics in my gut.

Ultimately, an abscessed tooth poisoned my body, resulting in ten medical diagnoses in the following order:

1. Depression
2. Bimonthly periods caused by uterine polyps
3. Ovarian cyst
4. Adrenal fatigue
5. Hormonal imbalance
6. Retinal tear
7. Visual migraines
8. Anemia
9. Low vitamin D level
10. Candidiasis infection of my colon

After my colonic therapist educated me about the candida overgrowth, I took an anti-candida cleanse and followed a strict anti-candida diet to get rid of this infection. I fought this culprit and restored my digestive flora with probiotics.

Killing the candida was a slow process, but I was determined to succeed because I desperately wanted to be well. Ultimately, I restored my adrenal glands and regained my energy. After eight months on the diet, I finally killed the *Candida* and regained my health.

God gave us glorious bodies that will heal themselves if we give them the right building blocks. Two years after the crown was placed on my tooth, I found this verse: "God is our merciful Father and the source of all comfort. He comforts us in all our troubles so that we can comfort others. When they are troubled, we will be able to give them the same comfort God has given us" (2 Corinthians 1:3–4).

My newfound purpose is to help you. I've experienced the devastating effects of being ill. Now I desire to help others reclaim their health as I did mine. A decade has passed since my illness, and now I am in my sixties. But I feel younger today than I did then. People tell me I look a decade younger too, and they want to know what I do to age gracefully. In this book, I share those ideas, along with their scientific foundations. I am a science geek and love to research ways to improve my brain, bones, and body so I look and feel younger. Now I share those secrets with you.

OUR JOURNEY TOGETHER

In *12 Ways to Age Gracefully*, we'll explore all aspects of our health—body, mind, and spirit. First, we'll discuss the foods to eat and avoid. We need to eat God's food and not processed, manufactured foodlike substances. You will learn accurate knowledge about today's food and discover how to tap into God's power to evoke lifestyle changes you may struggle to implement on your own.

The next chapter explains the importance of a balanced gastrointestinal tract—your gut. An unbalanced one decreases immunity and sets up the process of disease and overeating. Chapter 3 discusses the secret to stay physically active to maintain our body's vitality and how to modify exercise due to injuries, ailments, and disease. We must commit to exercising our bodies. Otherwise, our muscles and bones deteriorate. If we exercise, we feel more energetic and look younger. God gave us miraculous bodies, and we don't move them like we should. We sit, stand, and walk short distances. Those movements don't mobilize the spine enough. The more limber your spine, the younger you look. We feel better when we exercise.

I am especially interested in maintaining mental acuity in the senior years as my mother had dementia and my father-in-law suffered from Alzheimer's. In chapter 4, I provide the latest scientific research to prevent and improve these brain diseases.

We need to avoid environmental toxins, and chapter 5 shows you how. Stress and toxins wreak havoc on our health. Balanced hormones cause a person to be happier, so chapter 6 examines this topic. Did you know plastics disrupt our hormones? Yet most of our food is packaged in plastic.

We review stress reduction techniques in chapter 7. If we don't reduce our stress, our mental health can suffer. We'll examine these issues in chapter 8. Our emotional health is affected by many life events in later years, such as empty-nest syndrome, retirement, divorce, or loss of a spouse. Chapter 9 helps us adjust to these major life changes in healthy ways.

God created humans as complex beings who live in a social world. Our families, communities, and occupations are life components that we review in chapter 10. Since we're living longer these days, we can work longer. Instead of retiring in their sixties, some may choose to work well into their seventies. We may even need to work longer to afford our retirement years. Learn how to thrive with purpose in your senior years.

Our spiritual lives are another facet to our complexity, so we'll explore this side of a healthy life in chapter 11. We need to spend time with the Lord and be rooted in his Word. Change comes through the fruit of the spirit, which is given to us by the Holy Spirit. It is hard to make these lifestyle changes to improve our health. Tapping into God's power helps us reach our physical, spiritual, and emotional goals.

Finally, we wrap up with healthy habits in chapter 12 to balance all the aspects of your life. The first step to growing younger is making a choice. Decide and commit to caring for the body God gave you. This includes exercising almost every day of the week. This routine needs to become a habit. It takes sixty-three days to form a habit, not twenty-one, as many have said.[1] Your mind takes over two months to become deeply rooted in a new routine.

Aging seems inevitable. But is it? While we can't stop the clock, and each day does add length to our lives, the quality of our days can increase, not decrease, as the years go by. Most of us don't want to think about what will happen as we get into our seventies and eighties, especially if we don't care for ourselves. I did not want to cast the burden on my children of having to care for me in my senior years, so I worked on my total well-being after my health crises to improve the odds of having a healthy body and mind well into my nineties. We must make a commitment and develop healthy habits. Otherwise, our bodies will degenerate.

If you are healthy, you will live longer and can be a godly influence on the next generation. If you have grandchildren or great-grandchildren, you want to be around to teach them to be followers of Jesus Christ. You can't do that from the grave or hospital bed.

The decision to improve your health is personal. No one can make this decision for you; it is your choice. When you do, you will see encouraging results—a positive mindset, weight loss, decreased joint pain, fewer headaches, and improved energy. This book will help you change to birth a younger you.

You only have one body. If you do not care for it, you cannot fulfill your God-given mission. Make your body a priority every single day of your life. Take care of yourself physically, spiritually, mentally, and emotionally, so you will age gracefully.

CHAPTER 1

EAT TO LIVE LONGER

Thou shouldst eat to live; not live to eat.
—commonly attributed to Socrates

Given the creativity in packaging, labeling, and marketing of foods and meal plans today, figuring out what type of food to eat is confusing. Just because an item claims it contains natural ingredients or is gluten-free does not mean it is beneficial. Then there are the ads and anecdotal evidence for various eating plans. One person touts keto while another recommends a paleo diet. The high-fat Mediterranean diet is heart healthy, but low-fat diets were the rage in the 1980s. Talk about confusing. With so much contradictory information and the ads and stories everywhere on social media, how can you figure out the best diet?

When determining if a food is healthy or not, I use one simple motto—eat God's food. Look at your plate and determine if the food resembles produce from a garden or meat from a ranch. If it does, eat it. If the food item was shredded, dyed, and formed into a shape, do not eat it.

You do not need to count calories or measure your food. If you only eat what the Lord created and not the food manufacturers' concoctions, your health and weight will return to normal, naturally. You do not need to be concerned about counting calories because your body will take care of the rest.

Deciding what to eat for a healthy lifestyle does not have to be complicated. The following low-carb, low-sugar, anti-inflammatory eating guidelines are my secret to maintaining optimal weight and brain health. This type of diet improves memory and cognition while preventing and even reversing type 2 diabetes. It also decreases inflammation in the body.

Each person is different, but some foods may irritate a person's digestive tract and ultimately cause inflammation in other parts of the body. Three of the most common culprits are sugar, wheat, and dairy—we will discuss why later in this chapter. The top eight food allergens include eggs, fish, milk, nuts, peanuts, shellfish, soy, and wheat. If you are allergic to any of these foods or they cause abnormal symptoms (belching, gas, acid reflux, headache, foggy brain, joint pain), then they are most likely causing inflammation. Therefore, you should avoid these foods.

My personal low-carbohydrate, anti-inflammatory dietary guidelines include the following:

- Strive to make about 50 percent of your food items fresh, organic vegetables.
- Do not eat only cooked foods. Eat a couple of servings of raw vegetables every day. Have a salad for lunch with either nuts or meat. When eating out, order either a salad or coleslaw as a side since both are raw.
- Eat one fresh serving of low-glycemic fruit per day. These include green apples, berries, cherries, pears, plums, and grapefruit.
- Another 25 percent of your daily food intake should come from an animal or vegetable protein, such as beans, nuts, and lean meat. Fish is exceptionally nutritious. Try to eat it once a week.
- Eat a variety of raw nuts and seeds for an excellent source of protein, minerals, and essential fatty acids.
- Try not to consume anything containing more than ten grams of sugar in one serving.
- Avoid sugar, flour, and white rice. Instead, eat more fruits, vegetables, and low-glycemic grains, such as quinoa and pearled barley.
- Do not eat sugary cereals. Instead, prepare organic oatmeal, fruit, or granola. Be careful, as the sugar content of some granola choices may be high.

- Eat nontraditional grains, such as quinoa, amaranth, pearled barley, wild or brown rice, and organic oats to avoid gut problems that can come from wheat.
- Eat cultured foods, such as kimchi or sauerkraut, which contain natural probiotics. Add one to two tablespoons of these foods to a meal twice a week. And take a probiotic capsule daily.
- Replace fried foods with baked foods.
- Replace sugary snacks with nuts, nut butter, dark chocolate, and nondairy yogurt with berries.
- Replace condiments and sauces containing monosodium glutamate (MSG), high-fructose corn syrup, or sugar with no-sugar versions, spices, vinegar, and herbs.

Eating healthy foods all the time is unattainable, but if we strive to eat well 80 percent of the time, it is probably an improvement. Each morning as I wake up, my body tells me how well I ate the previous day. If I ate God's food and did not experience blood-sugar fluctuations, I have a clear mind and ample energy. The incredible sensation of how God created our bodies to feel motivates me to continue to eat well every day. I am more productive when I eat healthy foods.

Do you feel a difference when you eat high-carbohydrate or high-sugar foods? What symptoms do you experience? High-carb foods release glucose into the bloodstream and cause a corresponding rise in insulin. If we constantly tax our pancreas to release insulin, this organ wears out and type 2 diabetes ensues. Therefore, avoid the following high-carbohydrate foods: cakes, crackers, sugary cereals and drinks, flours, bread products, jellies/jams, and refined potato products. These types of foods are addictive.[1]

ORGANIC VERSUS NONORGANIC PRODUCE

Our bodies receive most environmental toxins through the foods we consume. Farmers spray produce with herbicides to kill the weeds growing around it and pesticides to stop the bugs from eating it. These chemicals are harmful to the human body. Should we purchase organic produce? That depends.

The nonprofit Environmental Working Group (EWG) is dedicated to protecting the environment and our health. That is why every spring, this Washington, DC–based advocacy group creates the Dirty Dozen and Clean Fifteen produce lists. They measure the pesticide residue left on fruit and vegetables after they have been washed and peeled. The Dirty Dozen list includes the varieties of produce that had the highest concentration of pesticides. Therefore, purchase organic fruits and vegetables from the list below:

- strawberries
- spinach
- kale, collard, and mustard greens
- peaches
- pears
- nectarines
- apples
- grapes
- bell and hot peppers
- cherries
- blueberries
- green beans[2]

The Clean Fifteen list is produce with the least amount of pesticide residue. You do not need to purchase organic produce from the list below:

- avocados
- sweet corn
- pineapple
- onions
- papaya
- sweet peas, frozen
- asparagus
- honeydew melon
- kiwi
- cabbage
- mushrooms
- mangoes
- sweet potatoes
- watermelon
- carrots[3]

The Dirty Dozen and Clean Fifteen lists help me determine which produce items to buy organic. If a thick-skinned vegetable is not on the Clean Fifteen list, you don't need to purchase organic. But if you eat the skin of the fruit and it is not on the clean list, buy organic.

CANCER-CAUSING CHEMICALS

A century ago, before manufacturers processed foods, fruits and vegetables grew on farms and were distributed to local regions. Fresh produce needed to be eaten quickly. Wheat was a whole grain and had a short shelf life. Today, manufacturers remove the bran and germ from the wheat kernel to extend the product's shelf life. Unfortunately, it doesn't contain the original nutrients. Many of today's processed foods don't resemble the original food they were made from and contain the herbicidal active ingredient glyphosate.

This carcinogenic weed-killing chemical, glyphosate, is sprayed on crops just prior to harvesting to help dry out the plant. Therefore, the chemical residue remains on the produce during harvest. Unfortunately, the federal government does not check for glyphosate residue on foods. Many countries around the world ban this toxic chemical.

In 2018, EWG assessed glyphosate levels in many grocery store oat products. Unfortunately, the EWG found glyphosate in every sample of popular oat-based cereal and food products.[4] Some items included granola, oatmeal, cereal, and snack bars. Unfortunately, these cereals are popular with children because they see the commercials on television. In some European countries, like Denmark, manufacturers are not allowed to market to children through commercials during children's television programs.

Since children have smaller bodies, they might absorb higher concentrations of glyphosate. Perhaps that is why, in the United States, cancer is the second leading cause of death in children five to nine years old.

To counteract the effects of glyphosate, the US agricultural industry has genetically modified four principal crops to be resistant to this herbicide.[5] These GMO foods are wheat, soy, corn, and sugar beets. Since these GMO crops are not harmed by glyphosate, they can be sprayed with it throughout the growing and harvesting season. Therefore, you could be consuming a carcinogen when you eat products made with these foods.[6]

In fact, in 2018 a San Francisco court ordered the food industry giant Monsanto to pay DeWayne Johnson $289 million in damages because glyphosate caused his cancer—non-Hodgkin's lymphoma.[7] Cancer is the second leading cause of death in the United States in adults as well. What we eat affects our risk of getting cancer.[8]

Many consumers are unaware that products made from oats, corn, wheat, soy, or sugar beets may contain the residue from a cancer-causing herbicide. Thousands of edible products are made from these five ingredients. Most of us feed our children dry cereal. Many foods with these ingredients contain sugar, which causes the consumer to eat more of it, as sugar may be an addictive substance to the body.

To avoid foods that contain glyphosate residue, purchase organic products made from corn, soy, wheat, oats, and sugar beets. According to the *Journal of the American Medical Association*, eating organic foods is strongly correlated with a dramatic reduction in cancer.[9] The article states, "Our results appear to suggest that promoting organic food consumption in the general population could be a promising preventive strategy against cancer."

Organic foods are not genetically modified (GMO), nor are they sprayed with pesticides or herbicides.[10] It may cost a little more for organic products, but poor health is much more expensive than healthy groceries.

As consumers, we need to be aware of the harmful by-products that may be on our foods. Our well-being and the health of our families is at stake. Food manufacturers are not consumer advocates because they need to make a profit. We can't always trust that the items on the grocery store shelf are safe.

BENEFICIAL FOODS

Figuring out which foods are beneficial versus harmful is difficult because of false and conflicting information. Be discerning about where you get your information and ensure that it is from a reputable source backed by scientific evidence.

Think of foods as being dead or alive. Food from a bag sitting on a grocery store shelf for months is dead and does not give your body the nutrients it needs to be healthy. However, a fresh salad is a live food that contains essential vitamins, minerals, and fiber the body needs.

Fiber in produce fills your stomach and tells your body you are full. When the fiber is removed from processed foods, it takes a larger quantity to fill you up. The fiber in fruit slows your digestion and reduces the effects of the natural sugar in the fruit, so your blood-sugar level does not rise as much.

As you eliminate processed foods from your diet, you should consume more whole, organic fruits, vegetables, whole grains (oats, brown rice, quinoa, barley), beans, nuts, seeds, fish, and meat. Your body will react positively to the nourishment and respond by healing. Look at each food and assess whether it is good for you. When you primarily eat dead food, you may be hungry more often, and your cells may not get the nutrients they need.

If a cell within the human body replicates incorrectly, it is called cancer. How can your body replace old cells with healthy new ones if you don't give it the essential vitamins and minerals it requires? This is especially important with aging.

Senescent cells are old human cells that stopped dividing but didn't die. The more old cells we have, the more we age. One of the most significant biological processes behind aging is an accumulation of senescent cells. These cells no longer function as they should; they are larger than normal and resistant to dying. They also secrete harmful inflammatory proteins that destroy or impair the function of healthy cells around them.[11]

Senescent cells accumulate with age. Removing senescent cells is critical to improving aging because they cause inflammation in the body. When these cells decrease, age-related chronic inflammation also decreases.[12]

Removing senescent cells reminds me of a facial. During the treatment, the aesthetician removes the old cells from the top layer of skin on the client's face. After the facial, the fresh new skin is moisturized and glowing. The client looks much younger.

To get rid of our aged cells, we need to eat God's food and occasionally fast. If we eat all the time, we do not allow our bodies the time and energy to repair cancerous cells and remove senescent cells.[13]

Autophagy is a natural way that the body gets rid of old cells, in order to create new ones. Unfortunately, autophagy decreases with age.[14] Dietary restriction or fasting increases the body's natural autophagy process, and so far, it is the most robust anti-aging therapy we can adopt.[15] Calorie-restricted diets reduced the aging process in lab animals. The animals became more active, suffered less from chronic diseases, and lived longer.[16] Dietary restrictions may help us to be more fit and live longer disease-free.

Research on senescent cell therapy started years ago at the Mayo Clinic. Their studies have shown that senescent cells negatively impact health and shorten life span by as much as 35 percent in normal mice.[17]

To rid your body of its old cells naturally, try intermittent fasting (giving your body at least twelve hours of no food overnight before breaking the fast—*breakfast*) or fast for one twenty-four-hour period once a week or every couple of weeks. Get your doctor's approval and advice before fasting.

We must be careful about what we put into our bodies because we receive the most toxins from what we eat. Try not to eat foods with more than five ingredients or ten grams of sugar per serving. The American Heart Association recommends limiting your calories from sugar. Women should consume no more than twenty-five grams of sugar or one hundred calories per day from sugar. Men should eat no more than thirty-six grams of sugar or one hundred fifty calories from sugar per day.[18]

Read food label ingredients to check for sugar, and if you can't pronounce an ingredient, it may be a food product your body won't recognize either. Begin to simplify the foods you consume. Eat foods closer to the form they were in when they came out of the garden. Ask yourself, "Did the food I am about to eat come out of the garden or off the ranch?"

Be aware of the food industry's marketing enticements that claim a product is natural or whole. It is far better to eat God's foods as close to harvest as possible when the nutritional value is the highest versus processed foods that have been stripped of the nutrients that benefit your body.

Good Veggies

About half of the food you consume should be organic vegetables. Maybe that's why the Lord created over one hundred vegetables to choose from. (I am classifying fruits and vegetables by nutritional and culinary standards, not botanical standards. That means I will call a tomato a vegetable and not a fruit.[19]) Let's look at only half the vegetables available on earth:

- acorn squash
- artichoke
- asparagus
- avocado
- beet
- bell pepper
- black bean
- black-eyed pea
- bok choy
- broad bean
- broccoli
- brussels sprout
- butternut squash
- cabbage
- carrot
- cauliflower
- celery
- chard
- chickpea or garbanzo
- collard green
- corn
- cucumber
- eggplant
- green bean
- kale
- kidney bean
- kohlrabi
- legume
- lettuce
- lentils
- lima bean or butter bean
- mustard green
- navy bean
- okra
- onion family
- parsnip
- pattypan squash
- peas
- peppers
- pinto bean
- potato
- pumpkin
- radish
- rhubarb
- rutabaga
- snap peas
- soybean
- spaghetti squash
- spinach
- sweet potato or yam
- tomato
- turnip
- yellow squash
- zucchini

Do you tend to eat the same vegetables all the time? Green beans, broccoli, and asparagus are my go-to veggies. Instead, it is better to vary the vegetables you eat. Try some new ones. They each contain different nutrients and ripen in different seasons. Eat what is ripe in a specific season: berries and spinach in the spring; tomatoes and peppers in the summer; butternut squash and pumpkin in the fall; and citrus fruits in the winter. God created different produce items to ripen seasonally to give us the nutrients we need in that season based upon what grows in your local area. Visit a farmer's market and pick up some fresh local produce harvested in that season.

Good Fruit

Check out this list of the variety of fruits the Lord created:

- apple
- apricot
- banana
- blueberry
- blackberry
- cantaloupe
- cherry
- cranberry
- currant
- date
- fig
- grape
- grapefruit
- guava
- honeydew melon
- kiwi
- kumquat
- lemon
- lime
- mango
- nectarine
- orange
- papaya
- peach
- pear
- persimmon
- pineapple
- plum
- pomegranate
- raspberry
- starfruit
- strawberry
- tangerine
- watermelon

Fruits are God's dessert. Eat them instead of a man-made dessert. Or make your own dessert using fruit. Berry cobbler is one of my favorites, and I use an alternative flour to bake it.

Good Grains

Again, the Lord gave us a variety of grains to consume, but we primarily eat one type—wheat. Instead, try these healthier grains that have not been modified and don't promote inflammation:

- amaranth
- barley
- buckwheat
- millet
- oats
- quinoa
- rice
- rye
- wild rice

Replace your processed white rice with whole grain rice.

Good Nuts

Nuts are a great source of protein. I take a bag of nuts along when I attend ball games, go hiking, or travel. No refrigeration needed. Do you eat any of these nuts?

- almond
- Brazil
- cashew
- chestnut
- hazelnut
- macadamia
- pecan
- pistachio
- pine nut
- walnut

Getting locally sourced nuts through a farmers market or farm is the least expensive and most nutritious way to obtain them. Raw nuts are best because their nutritional value is intact and has not been altered by roasting. Pecans grow in my area, so I get a year's worth annually from a local farmer. I store those pecans in quart mason jars in the freezer.

Good Seeds

Seeds contain trace minerals that our body needs. Try eating some of these:

- chia
- flax
- hemp
- poppy
- pumpkin
- sesame
- sunflower

I add hemp, sesame, and sunflower seeds to salads. Add ground flax seeds to oatmeal. For a healthy, delicious breakfast, add one-third cup of water to two tablespoons of chia seeds to make a chia seed pudding. Wait ten minutes for the seeds to plump up and add all sorts of fruit, seeds, and nuts to the mixture.

Shopping for Good Foods

When grocery shopping, primarily shop along the edges of the store in the produce, meat, and refrigerated sections. Stay away from the center of the store where processed foods are located. These products have an extended shelf life. Apparently they must not contain as many nutrients as fresh produce, which spoils.

This change in your diet may feel radical and seem limiting, but God gave us an incredible variety of food to enjoy and sustain our bodies, including over one hundred vegetables and fruits. You want to eat from God's food groups–vegetables, fruits, meats, nuts, seeds, and grains (excluding modern wheat). Many of the health problems we suffer start with unhealthy eating habits. You can change your life by changing the types of food you eat.

FOODS TO AVOID

Now that we've discussed what to eat, we want to understand what not to eat. Delectable yet unhealthy foods are easily available, and often appear less expensive. Yet our health is worth investing in. If we know which products are damaging to our bodies, we can avoid them. Let's look at the list of foods to avoid.

Wheat

I do not recommend eating any foods containing wheat because today's wheat is hybridized, and therefore, is not the same healthy grain that humans ate for centuries. Modern wheat is dwarf and drought-resistant. I believe this new form of wheat created in the 1950s caused the high level of gluten sensitivity we see today. Fifty years ago, gluten intolerance was rare.

I think the gluten in the hybrid wheat changed so much that it became more difficult to digest, causing some individuals to become sensitive or intolerant to the gluten. In fact, older varieties of wheat, such as einkorn and emmer, may be better tolerated by those with a gluten-related condition than the current strains used in food production.

For centuries, people flourished by consuming bread, but since wheat is not the same today as it was then, avoid wheat-based products. No bagels, waffles, pancakes, cake, muffins, pizza, pretzels, pasta—the list goes on and on. However, a great selection of gluten-free products is now available to replace these food items we are accustomed to eating. But make sure your gluten-free products are not made with white rice flour as that is high in carbs.

To find out if you are gluten-sensitive, either take the gluten quiz at GlutenIntoleranceQuiz.com or fast from gluten for a whole month. This length of time is necessary because the gluten molecule is so large it may take weeks before the body can eliminate it. As you reintroduce gluten back into your diet, note any adverse side effects such as bloating, diarrhea, gas, smelly feces, constipation, nausea, vomiting, abdominal pain, headache, foggy mind, joint pain, nasal congestion, depression, fatigue, skin problems, and autoimmune diseases.

Wheat is one of the top eight allergenic foods. If a person's body does not recognize gluten as food, their immune system attacks the gluten and, unfortunately, their body at the same time. This causes inflammation, and inflammation promotes aging.

Processed foods, like white flour, do not go bad because food manufacturers removed the natural nutrients to extend the shelf life.[20] The milling process for flour production involves removing the bran and germ from wheat kernels, leaving mostly the endosperm. This is because the bran and germ contain fats that can cause the flour to go rancid, thus reducing its shelf life. During milling, these parts are separated out to produce a more stable product that lasts longer on the shelf. However, this also removes many of the nutrients found in whole wheat. To address the nutrient loss, flour is often enriched by adding back certain vitamins and minerals that were present before processing.

This benefits companies' bottom lines but is detrimental to our health. If we eat processed foods that do not contain nutrients, we deprive ourselves of essential vitamins and minerals. A lack of nutrients leads to malnutrition, which promotes disease and aging. We consume products made from white flour all the time. Maybe that is why over 60 percent of Americans experience chronic diseases.[21] This staggering statistic is not shared by European countries.

If you choose to eat organic wheat, or any type of grain, make sure it is sprouted. Grains have an enzyme that inhibits the release of our digestive enzymes. Therefore, grains are harder to digest than other foods, and remain in our intestines too long, which creates a bloated belly. Soaking grains in water breaks down the enzyme inhibitor and improves their digestibility. Proper digestion of food is vital to absorb the nutrients.[22]

White Rice

To extend the shelf life of rice, food manufacturers remove the husk, bran, and germ from the rice during the milling process.[23] Since most of the grain's nutrients are removed, it has a long shelf life. Therefore, white rice is processed and raises blood-sugar levels.

Taking the beneficial nutrients out of food is not how God intended for us to eat. The Lord created *whole* grains for our body to assimilate all the nutrients and fiber. Fiber keeps the bowels moving smoothly. Consuming brown and wild rice is fine because they contain the whole grain of the rice including the fiber and nutrients. Again, make sure the rice is sprouted.

Sugar

Sugar-sweetened drinks raise blood-sugar levels. To counteract the high blood-sugar level, the pancreas releases insulin, which then causes blood-sugar levels to plummet. The resulting symptoms are lethargy and irritability.

Sugar and wheat are addictive, and they comprise a large part of the American diet. These products cause the release of dopamine from the same brain receptors as opiate drugs.[24] On a Positron Emission Tomography Scan (PET) of the human brain, the same area of the brain lit up when an obese person ingested sugar and an addict received cocaine.[25] Many Americans are addicted to sugar and carbohydrates. These products contribute to diseases and obesity.

Many grocery store items such as yogurt, ketchup, salad dressings, cereals, soups, and drinks contain hidden sources of sugar. Even nut butters may have sugar added to them. Why? Maybe food manufacturers want us to buy more of their products.

Substitute sugar with a natural sweetener. One example is stevia, which is an herb. Make sure the stevia you purchase does not contain dextrose or other forms of sugar. Another option is local honey. However, use honey sparingly as it raises blood-sugar levels. Monk fruit is another natural sweetener with zero calories that rates zero on the glycemic index (which measures how the food increases your blood sugar level). The following list ranks natural sugar substitutes based on their glycemic index:[26]

- stevia – 0
- monk fruit sweetener – 0
- xylitol – 12
- agave – 15
- coconut sugar – 35
- honey – 50
- maple syrup – 54

Choose a natural, low-glycemic sweetener you can live with and use it sparingly.

Corn

Unfortunately, most of the corn in the United States has been genetically modified (GMO) to be resistant to herbicides. Herbicidal proteins were put into the genetically engineered seed. Corn with herbicidal proteins allows the plant to tolerate glyphosate—the carcinogenic chemical found in many herbicides.[27]

Farmers can spray the GMO corn with herbicides, and as a result, we consume corn with a carcinogenic residue. I do not recommend eating corn unless it is organic. Make sure your corn tortilla chips and popcorn are organic, as well as any other product made from corn.

Milk Products

There is a lot of debate over whether pasteurized milk or raw milk is better for you. There are pluses and minuses on both sides. If you choose to consume dairy, do your own research and decide what is best for you and your family.

I recommend consuming almond, cashew, coconut, or organic oat milk products instead of dairy. I eat coconut milk ice cream, and I can't taste much difference between the cow or coconut milk products.

Corn Syrup

High-fructose corn syrup (HFCS) is an inexpensive alternative to sugar that was introduced to the American food system in the late 1970s. This product keeps food manufacturing costs down. There are many differing opinions on the use of HFCS in the food industry. Depending on the source, HFCS has a glycemic index of anywhere between 50 and 73.[28] The increased use of this product may partially account for the rapid increase in obesity in the United States.[29]

Artificial Sweeteners

I do not recommend artificial sweeteners. Food manufacturers make these sweeteners in a lab. Instead, use God's sweeteners such as stevia, honey, maple syrup, agave, coconut sugar, or monk fruit sugar. Those who consume man-made sugar substitutes may have a higher risk of gaining weight.[30] Diet sodas contain artificial sweeteners. Unfortunately, many people think they are being healthy by substituting diet drinks for sugary drinks, but they are not.

Processed Meats

Processed meats (hot dogs, ham, bacon, sausage, and some deli meats) were classified as a group 1 carcinogen by the World Health Organization.[31] Tobacco, asbestos, and plutonium are also listed as group 1 carcinogens. I feel terrible about how many hot dogs I fed my kids.

Meat processing includes salting, fermenting, curing, and smoking. Avoid purchasing any prepackaged lunch meats. Instead, use baked chicken as lunch meat. If you buy meat at a deli, make sure the attendant cuts slices from a hunk of meat that came from an animal versus the meat being shredded and formed into a mold. For instance, if chicken parts are processed together into a molded, premade, unnatural patty, they are unhealthy.

Vegetable Oils

Vegetable oils that contain omega-6 fatty acids, such as corn and soy oil, may promote inflammation in the body.[32] Therefore, we should lower our consumption of omega-6 foods and increase our ingestion of omega-3 foods (which nourish the brain[33]) like avocado, nuts, and fish. Olive oil is the preferred oil to use because it contains both omega-3 and -6 fats and is high in antioxidants.[34] But olive oil should be used at lower temperatures, not on high heat, so its beneficial properties don't break down.

Coconut oil is another beneficial oil, and it resists oxidation at high heat. Use coconut oil for high-heat cooking, such as frying. Coconut oil also reduces triglycerides, LDL, and total cholesterol levels.[35] Avocado oil is another alternative. Buy cold-pressed oils in glass jars because plastic containers can leach into the oil.

Processed Foods

Processed foods have been stripped of their God-given nutrients to extend their shelf life. You will find them in boxes and bags in the grocery store aisles. Processed foods are dead foods that do not benefit the body but instead harm it. Do not eat any processed foods, including cereals, chips, crackers, cookies, and so on.

We can't eat perfectly all the time. For example, we may be a guest for dinner at someone's home. If you choose to eat processed food, make sure it is organic and non-GMO. Eat to live a healthy, bountiful life. Evaluate every single thing you eat. Is it alive or dead? Remember, shelf life means no life.

Peanuts

Peanuts are not a nut but a legume (that is, a pea or bean). They don't grow on a tree but grow in the ground. I do not recommend consuming peanut butter because some people find it hard to digest, and many people are allergic to it.

I live near a peanut field. The peanuts are dug up and left on the ground to dry for a couple of weeks. During that time, they get soaked from rain, and I can only imagine how much mold may grow on them in the humid Florida weather. Almond or cashew butters are better choices.

Canned Goods

Many canned foods are lined with Bisphenol A (BPA) to prevent erosion of the can. BPA is an industrial chemical used to make some plastics. An ongoing debate ensues between scientific studies and the Federal Drug Administration (FDA) regarding whether the level of BPA found in canned foods is safe for humans.[36] Unfortunately, when we eat canned foods, we are exposed to this chemical.

The FDA banned the use of certain BPA-based materials used in infant bottles, sippy cups, and infant formula packaging.[37] What does that tell you about its safety? Therefore, do not eat foods from cans. Food preserved in glass (such as spaghetti sauce), not cans, is a better option.

Margarine

Most likely margarine contains trans fat, which increases the risk of heart disease and free radicals, thus contributing to numerous health problems, including cancer. Instead, use organic butter, olive oil, and coconut oil.

You may be surprised about the list of foods you should avoid. However, these foods cause inflammation in your body. That is why your joints ache, and you feel lousy. If you remove the inflammatory-promoting foods, you remove the root cause of many health issues. I believe in resolving the source versus treating the symptom with a drug. Replace the foods listed above with vegetables, fruits, nuts, seeds, meats, or sprouted grains, excluding wheat. Eat until you are full. This is not a diet but a lifestyle change to promote health through eating God's food. Simply changing the types of food you eat can help you age gracefully.

SUPPLEMENTATION

Our soil today does not contain the nutrients it did a century ago before the Industrial Revolution and big-time agricultural farming.[38] Because micronutrients are no longer in our soil and foods, many of us need to supplement to ensure we receive all the nutrients the body needs to function optimally.

Nutrients are like fertilizer for your body and brain. Many people are low on their daily needs for several vitamins, such as vitamin D and B12. Ask your physician to test your levels to see if you need to supplement with these vitamins. (However, if your levels are normal, you do not need to supplement them. Discuss it with your doctor. It is possible to have too much of a good thing.) If your levels are low, I recommend the following supplements:

- multivitamin
- mineral supplement
- vitamin D, if your level is not optimum
- vitamin B12, if your level is low or you eat little meat
- magnesium
- probiotics (addressed in chapter 2)

Most people need a superior multivitamin that includes zinc. Since I suffered from adrenal fatigue a decade ago, I still take a high-powered multivitamin recommended for adrenal health, along with an accompanying vitamin C supplement.

Calcium and potassium are vital minerals that should be included in your multimineral supplement. If you take calcium, take it along with vitamin K because too much calcium can cause unwanted calcium deposits in the body, but vitamin K helps prevent this.[39]

I purchase mineral supplements like I do my probiotics—I buy a different brand each time the bottle is empty. Many microminerals are available, so I switch around what I take. I credit my minimal graying hair color to this powerful supplementation. A National Institutes of Health study concluded, "Premature graying may be an indicator that hair is not getting enough nutrients and minerals, and supplementation with these trace elements might reverse and is expected to prevent progression."[40]

Vitamin D deficiency is a common worldwide problem. This vitamin helps our bodies absorb and use calcium and phosphorus to build bones, which helps prevent osteoporosis. Symptoms of low vitamin D are fatigue, muscle weakness/aches/cramps, bone pain, and mood changes like depression.[41] We absorb this vitamin through our skin when we get twenty minutes of sun daily without sunscreen. Most of us do not get that much sun, so we need to supplement.

Normal vitamin D blood test levels differ from lab to lab but generally are 30–72 nanograms per milliliter (ng/mL). My sister's vitamin D level was 36, and her physician told her that was normal. Yes, the level was within the normal range, but it was not optimal. When my level was that low, I was tired all the time. When I increased my level above 50 ng/mL, my energy improved. Make sure your vitamin levels are optimal for you and not just on the low side of normal.

Vitamin B12 deficiencies are more common in people who do not eat much meat and in seniors because the ability to absorb vitamins from food declines with age.[42] Some common low B12 symptoms include fatigue, headaches, depression, and concentration difficulties.[43] Get your levels checked and supplement if needed.

Around half of Americans are deficient in magnesium. The Recommended Dietary Allowance for magnesium is 400 to 420 mg daily.[44] Symptoms of low magnesium are nausea, twitching or muscle cramping, frequent headaches, irregular heartbeat, weakness, and constipation.[45] After extreme physical exercise, I take a bath with magnesium flakes versus Epsom salts because the magnesium is more easily absorbed. Whatever bath salts you use, make sure they do not contain unnatural scents because you may absorb them, and this is one more item your body needs to detoxify.

Eating organic food is the best thing you can do to ensure you get the nutrients you need. Eating five produce items per day is recommended, but this is difficult to do. I take Juice Plus+ supplements because they bridge the gap between what I eat and what I may be lacking in my diet. Juice Plus+ capsules contain dehydrated fruits, berries, and vegetables, which help me meet the goal of eating five fruits and vegetables per day.

Get back the nutrients you've lost because of poor soil, environmental toxins, and the aging process. Eat God's foods and use supplementation, and you will lower your toxic burden and slow the progression of aging.

PERSONAL AND PRACTICAL APPLICATION

1. From the low-carbohydrate, anti-inflammatory dietary guidelines provided in this chapter, what can you do to improve your diet?
2. What produce items do you normally eat that are on the Dirty Dozen list?
3. How can you simplify the foods you eat?
4. When you are about to eat, ask yourself, "Does the food I am about to eat come from a garden or a ranch? Did God originally create this food?" Try this for a few days. What results did you discover?
5. Do you seem to eat the same vegetables all the time? What new produce items could you purchase?
6. On your next grocery shopping trip, check the sugar content to see if extra sugar was added to a product you normally purchase. What new insights did you find?
7. Have you ever thought of foods as being dead or alive? What dead foods have you eaten in the past twenty-four hours? What dead foods can you eliminate from your diet?
8. Can you feel a difference when you eat high-carbohydrate or high-sugar foods? What symptoms do you experience? (Try keeping a food diary for a few days to see how certain foods make you feel. Check out my book *Healthy Living Journal* if you are interested in keeping a food log.)
9. What changes do you plan to make in your diet based on the information from this chapter?
10. What supplements do you currently take? Do you think you should take any additional vitamins or minerals?

CHAPTER 2
KEEP YOUR GUT HEALTHY

A healthy outside starts from the inside.
—Robert Urich

"I knew it in my gut." "I need to trust my gut." "My gut tells me . . ." We often refer to our gut as a center of our instincts and our internal, personal guidance in spiritual and emotional decisions. Yet our actual physical gut is, in fact, the center of our physical well-being. Inflammation of our gut is the root of many illnesses. To age well, we must start making healthy choices from the inside out.

As you learn what you should and should not eat, you need to understand your digestive tract—the system that takes that food and distributes it to the rest of the body. If the food is not healthy, our gut will tell us. Many of us experience belching, gas, and acid reflux but ignore those symptoms as if they are normal. Those symptoms are *not* normal. Taking an ongoing medication to relieve nagging digestive issues is undesirable because it's not natural and doesn't get to the root of the problem. Instead of treating the symptoms, we should work on balancing our digestive tract.

If your gut is not healthy, you are not healthy. Once you heal your gut, it will be much easier to control your appetite. This secret will help you implement the chapter 1 nutritional guidelines.

GUT MICROBIOME

The gastrointestinal (GI) microbiome is a delicate balance of beneficial and potentially harmful bacteria, viruses, and yeast. The collection of microbes in your intestinal tract protects you when an attacker (bacteria, viruses, and allergens) tries to invade your body. If you have a healthy gut, you get sick less often.

The microbiome is part of the immune system that defends against bad microorganisms. A National Institutes of Health–funded study concluded, "The gut microbiota has a profound effect on the host immune system and can affect autoimmune-related diseases both within and outside the gut."[1] Some of those diseases include irritable bowel syndrome, rheumatoid arthritis, and systemic lupus erythematosus, but many types of autoimmune diseases can attack the body.[2]

In the past twenty years, the microbiome has become a highly active area of research because of the GI tract's importance to a person's overall health. When the bad guys inside your gut grow beyond normal limits, your microbiome becomes imbalanced (dysbiosis). This may cause digestive problems such as stomach pain, bloating, diarrhea, or constipation, in addition to autoimmune-related diseases. Moodiness, anxiety, and depression are also associated with dysbiosis.[3] The world inside your gastrointestinal tract affects many parts of your body.

You can improve your microbiome when you eat probiotic-rich foods or supplements, avoid processed and high-sugar foods, and eat the foods that God gave us—fresh vegetables, fruits, meats, sprouted whole grains, nuts, and seeds close to their form after harvest.[4] You have the power to balance your microbiome so that your body functions well.

Harmful Gut Microbes

Twice in my life, my digestive tract harbored harmful bacteria. The symptoms of both infections were minor—belching and craving carbs. I experienced no gastrointestinal distress.

How does a person know if they have a harmful bug in their gut? Stool tests diagnose unfriendly microbes. Most people haven't had such a test because physicians rarely order it unless you are showing symptoms of a parasitic infection. Harmful bacteria other than parasites can inhabit your GI tract.

If a person exhibits symptoms of an ulcer, severe gastrointestinal distress, or bleeding, then a doctor orders a colonoscopy or upper

GI series. However, a simple, noninvasive stool analysis provides a portrayal of an individual's gut health (microbiome). So why aren't noninvasive stool analyses performed more frequently as part of a preventive checkup, just like a blood test?

Last year, my functional medicine practitioner ordered a stool test called a Gastrointestinal Microbial Assay Plue (GI-MAP). This test checked for the following:

- parasites
- harmful bacteria, viruses, and yeast (*Candida*)
- bacteria that may trigger an autoimmune disease
- normal beneficial microorganisms
- gluten sensitivity
- gastrointestinal secretory gland functioning (how well you digest food)

My results revealed that a harmful bacterium, *Helicobacter pylori* (H. pylori), inhabited my digestive tract. H. pylori is a common bacterium that over half of the population has but does not know it.[5] For years, this bacterium can live in your body before you exhibit symptoms (bloating, burping, nausea, heartburn, and sometimes ulcers). The only symptom I had was burping after meals—that's it. If you don't experience symptoms, your doctor will probably not test you for it. You can have a breath test to check for H. pylori too. Ultimately, H. pylori could lead to gastric cancer, so it is vital to get this bug out of your gut.[6]

My doctor recommended an over-the-counter holistic medicine to kill the bacteria, which did not work. She then prescribed a triple treatment with two antibiotics and a protein pump inhibitor. It was tough taking these three medications for two weeks, but I knew I needed to get rid of this dangerous microbe.

The problem with antibiotics is that they kill both harmful and beneficial gut bacteria. Therefore, during and after the treatment I took three probiotic supplements, a different one each day, to reinoculate my digestive tract. I also ate sauerkraut because you can't get all your probiotics from a supplement; some must come from fermented food.

Three months after the treatment, my doctor repeated the GI-MAP stool analysis and found no H. pylori bacteria. After a couple months, my belching went away too.

Candida Overgrowth

Besides H. pylori, I've also experienced an overgrowth of candida. Two of the primary microorganisms that live inside your digestive tract are probiotics and a yeast called *Candida albicans*.[7] God created our bodies with the perfect balance between these microbes, so they live harmoniously in our guts. Unfortunately, many products in our foods harm this delicate balance. Many processed foods contain dyes, chemicals, excess sugar, and the residue of pesticides and herbicides, which can disrupt the gut equilibrium. However, the primary culprit of this imbalance is antibiotics. They kill beneficial microorganisms and cause a bad guy—*Candida*—to overgrow.[8]

Though I am a nurse, I was never taught to take probiotics while taking antibiotics and continue them for a month or two afterward. When antibiotics kill off the good microbes (probiotics), the *Candida* takes over. *Candida* yeast releases microtoxins in the body that wreak havoc on your health.[9] Therefore, it is critical to reculture your gut with probiotics.

One natural treatment method for a *Candida* infection is a diet that limits sugar, gluten, and alcohol. Many people believe you can starve *Candida*. Therefore, if you crave sugar, alcohol, and/or processed foods, you might have an imbalance in the flora of your gut. An imbalance (dysbiosis) means the helpful microorganisms have been killed off. The destruction of these beneficial microorganisms allows the harmful microbe *Candida* to multiply.[10]

Candida can become a fungal overgrowth in the lining of your gastrointestinal system, which can create intestinal permeability, also known as leaky gut. The permeability may allow leakage of substances from the gut into the body. Our bodies don't recognize these particles, so our immune system creates antibodies that cause food allergies and autoimmune diseases to develop.[11] Do you suffer from a food allergy or an autoimmune disease?

When *Candida* spreads and takes over your digestive tract, it acts like a parasite sucking the life and energy out of you. It is hard to fight the yeast's never-ending appetite for sugar, carbs, or alcohol. I had an overgrowth of *Candida*, so I know how hard it is to fight this offender. Every night, I couldn't stop my cravings for chocolate and red wine.

I created a quiz at CandiQuiz.com to help people determine if they may suffer from this issue. I don't want this bug to wreak havoc on your health like it did mine.

My Candida Infection

An abscessed tooth caused my ten medical diagnoses, including the *Candida* infection in my colon. Despite being a nurse, I had never heard of candidiasis (infection from a *Candida* fungus). Even my internal medicine doctor didn't know how to treat this yeast infection.

Consumed antibiotics and a steroid for my abscessed tooth killed the probiotics in my gut, so the *Candida* overgrew. Anyone could have candidiasis and not know it.

The most effective way to kill a *Candida* overgrowth is with a *Candida* cleanse and an anti-*Candida* diet—low carbohydrates and low sugar. Eating an organic paleo diet (meat, produce, nuts, and seeds) decreases the toxic load in a person's body. Just by eating in this manner your microbiome becomes more balanced.[12]

I ate this diet for eight months. I also took large doses of probiotics (up to 100 billion units/day) to provide my gut with the good microbes that had been destroyed.

Candida even began infecting my nails. Do you have hard, thick toenails? This is a sign of *Candida* infecting the nail bed. I remember my brother, who was an alcoholic, had a thick, discolored, and disfigured toenail. Now I understand it was from the *Candida* fungus.[13] The more times in your life you have taken antibiotics without replenishing your gastrointestinal tract with probiotics, the more likely you are to have a *Candida* overgrowth. Ultimately, I killed the *Candida* in my colon by taking the *Candida* cleanse and eating a strict low-carb diet.

Heal Your Gut

Do you burp, expel gas, suffer from stomachaches or heartburn? Do you pass abnormal stools? (Normal stools pass easily and are not watery.) These symptoms are not normal, but many people have grown used to them. When your microbiome is unbalanced, an array of conditions may occur, including autoimmune diseases.[14]

In November 2020, the media announced the following news release: "Link Between Alzheimer's Disease and Gut Microbiota Is Confirmed."[15] A study established the correlation between an imbalance in the gut microbiota and the development of amyloid plaques—the pathological sign of Alzheimer's disease. Who would have thought our gastrointestinal tract affected our brain? Our body is interconnected, and one part affects the other.

Researchers found that Alzheimer's patients had an altered (imbalanced) gut microbiome with fewer diverse probiotics, plus harmful gut bacteria. Harmful intestinal bacteria can trigger an inflammatory phenomenon in the body. You don't want this, so care for your gut before amyloid plaques develop in the brain. Improve your intestinal microbiome through probiotics. A doctor can help you kill the harmful gut bacteria.

As mentioned before, a simple, noninvasive stool analysis provides a portrayal of an individual's gut health (microbiome). Antibiotics, an overgrowth of *Candida*, undiagnosed gluten sensitivity, and a sugar-laden diet with loads of processed foods harm the intestinal tract's intricate balance. Follow these five steps to help heal your gut and balance its microbiome.

1. Eat a healthy low-sugar diet full of fresh vegetables and fruits, organic meats, nuts, seeds, and avoid grains. You want all of your food to come from the farm or ranch and not be processed. Outsmart the food manufacturers and get back to eating God's foods.

When my daughter was diagnosed with leaky gut syndrome and food sensitivities to eggs, soy, gluten, and dairy, her practitioner recommended a paleo diet, which excluded grains, dairy, and legumes. Wheat (gluten), dairy, and soy are three of the most common food allergens. If you currently experience gut issues, try eliminating these three food culprits from your diet for three to four weeks. Monitor whether or not your symptoms are relieved. A few weeks later, add them into your diet one at a time, checking to see if your symptoms return.

A person's GI tract may become permeable because of a *Candida* overgrowth and this is closely linked to food sensitivities.[16] Broken-down food particles can then enter the bloodstream and cause additional food allergies. It is not surprising that gluten sensitivity is often paired with an autoimmune condition because the body accidentally harms its own cells as it attacks the food it is sensitive to.

2. Figure out if you have a food sensitivity. Many of my health and wellness-coaching clients who experience chronic diarrhea have gluten sensitivity. Once they remove gluten from their diet, this annoying symptom disappears. If you want to understand why gluten-related disorders have increased by 400 percent in the last sixty years, read my book *Solving the Gluten Puzzle*. A doctor can order a blood test to check for food sensitivities.

3. Purchase digestive enzymes from a health food store and take them right before eating. As we age and unintentionally harm our gut microbiome's perfect balance, our stomachs do not produce as much hydrochloric acid.[17] Therefore, we need to help our bodies properly digest foods by supplementing with digestive enzymes. When food is not digested properly, we cannot absorb the nutrients from it.

If you eat meat, it is best to take a digestive enzyme that contains betaine hydrochloride. When our stomachs don't secrete sufficient amounts of hydrochloric acid, the undigested food promotes the growth of unwanted microbes and can create inflammation within the body. Digestive enzymes containing betaine hydrochloride help the stomach digest food properly, so the undigested food doesn't become a petri dish for bacteria.[18]

4. Add probiotics to your diet through food and supplements. Continue to repeat this for up to a year. I recommend taking a probiotic that contains at least ten billion active cultures from at least ten different strains. To get a wide range of beneficial microorganisms, I change the brand of my probiotic every time I purchase a new bottle. I also recommend eating probiotic-rich foods, such as sauerkraut and kimchi. Eating a tablespoon a couple of times a week is all you need.

Yogurts do not provide enough probiotics. I ate Greek nondairy yogurt several days a week and had a stool test that showed my probiotic level from food was low. A year later, after adding sauerkraut to my diet, my stool test showed a normal probiotic level in my gut that came from food. Most people do not enjoy sauerkraut, but you only need a small amount to get a sufficient quantity of beneficial probiotic microorganisms.

I do not recommend kefir or kombucha because both are high in sugar. I used to make my own kombucha by feeding loads of sugar to a SCOBY (**S**ymbiotic **c**ulture **o**f **b**acteria and **y**east, or more simply, a glob of yeast). Each week I made a new batch, and the SCOBY grew larger, just like it does when it overgrows in the GI tract. *Candida* thrives on sugars, and the sugar used in the fermentation of kombucha could potentially feed *Candida* yeast, exacerbating an overgrowth. Moreover, since kombucha also contains various yeast strains, there's a possibility that it may contribute to *Candida* proliferation if the strains are not beneficial. I've seen advertisements touting the probiotic benefits of the drink. This is an example of how confusing it is to differentiate harmful versus beneficial foods.

Ever since my illness and suffering from candidiasis, I have been more susceptible to a *Candida* overgrowth and an imbalance in my gut. That's why I still take a probiotic several times a week. When I crave sugar, carbs, or alcohol, I know the *Candida* is growing again. I may need to take proactive steps to stop its growth by decreasing my sugar intake and taking an anti-*Candida* cleanse.

5. To improve the integrity of the lining of the digestive tract, take an over-the-counter supplement called L-glutamine. This odorless, tasteless powder or capsule taken twice daily can heal the lining of the GI tract.[19] I add a scoop to a glass of water in the morning. I can't taste it. This supplement helps heal the stomach's secretory glands so you can produce more gastric enzymes to help with food digestion and kill harmful bacteria.

As health care consumers, we need to be more proactive with our medical practitioners regarding strategies to prevent diseases. We do not want to be part of the Centers for Disease Control statistics that show 60 percent of Americans suffer from a chronic disease and 42 percent experience obesity.[20]

Root Causes of Overeating

I believe in determining the root cause of a health issue versus treating the symptom. If you can resolve the issue that caused the problem, then you won't need medication for the symptoms. If you typically overeat or can't stop binging, explore what might be the root cause. Some causes include

- a lack of knowledge regarding bad foods like wheat,
- an overgrowth of *Candida* in the gastrointestinal tract,
- addiction to food,
- emotional connection to food, and
- stress eating.

To get healthy, you must find the root cause of your overeating. Instead of treating symptoms with a trendy diet, determine your negative issue with food and take steps to resolve it.

This book provides the knowledge you need to motivate yourself to change. But your health will only improve if you put that knowledge into practice. Once you've taken steps to relieve a *Candida* infection, next you need to address any unhealthy eating habits. Research has indicated that the daily intake of sugar can lead to a consistent release of dopamine in the brain's reward center, which can create a pattern similar to what is seen with addictive substances.[21] Dopamine makes you feel good. The way to solve the temptation to eat foods high in sugar is to remove them from your home and never buy them again.

Use scripture verses to help fight the overwhelming desire to consume an item you don't want to eat. I've placed the following verse on my refrigerator and pantry, "Don't drink too much wine, for many evils lie along that path; be filled instead with the Holy Spirit and controlled by him" (Ephesians 5:18 TLB). Replace the word *wine* with any food item to which you are addicted.

If you need support with breaking the sugar habit, please join my private Facebook group "7 Steps to Get Off Sugar, Carbs, and Gluten" and check out my bestseller *7 Steps to Get Off Sugar and Carbohydrates*.[22] Once you eliminate sugar, you will develop an aversion to it, believe it or not. Items you ate before will taste too sweet because your God-given palate will return. You will prefer to eat God's provision versus the food manufacturers'. You will naturally lose weight, and unwanted symptoms will subside.

Also, understand that you can release dopamine naturally through other activities. Exercise by walking around the neighborhood or do some jumping jacks. Turn on praise music and start singing. Singing releases many positive neurohormones.[23] Hug your grandchild or loved one and feel that joyful release. Write the positive things you can do instead of eating and put that list on your refrigerator—front and center. Read this list and recite your Bible verse out loud to fight temptation. You can overcome a food addiction.

An emotional connection with food is hard to break. That is why I wrote *Christian Study Guide for 7 Steps to Get Off Sugar and Carbohydrates*. I believe you have to mobilize God's power to evoke lifestyle changes you are unable to handle on your own. Use God's tactics of prayer, accountability, and Bible verses to fight the Enemy. He provides the Holy Spirit to give us the power to live a healthy and godly life.

Stress makes people crave high-carb, sugary comfort foods. These processed foods give you a sugar rush, but then your blood sugar crashes, and you feel rotten. If you understand the connection between stress and eating habits, you can be proactive. Instead of grabbing the bag of chips, grab a healthy food choice like nuts covered with dark chocolate. Exercise helps relieve stress. Add exercise to your weekly calendar so you will do it.

When you get to the root cause of dysfunctional eating issues, you can heal. If you don't, you get on the circuitous loop of gaining weight, dieting, losing weight, going off the diet, and regaining weight. This will age you faster and, in the long term, will keep you from feeling good the older you get. Stop the cycle. Figure out the root cause for overeating and work on resolving it. Choose to eat healthy foods for the rest of your life. You are not going on a diet but changing your food choices and creating a healthier lifestyle and longer life.

HOW TO LOSE WEIGHT

Many people ask me how to shed a few pounds. When I began eating in a healthy fashion, I saw how my weight and the balance of my body fat and muscle became healthier. I felt like a new woman. A few simple changes in your eating habits can help you lose a pound or two a week. In ten weeks, the weight loss adds up significantly. The following five healthy living tips will help you lose weight naturally without going on a diet.

1. Stop eating wheat. Yes, you heard me correctly. The primary "wheat" ingredient in most processed goods is white flour, which has been stripped of its God-given nutrients. That is why it can sit on the grocery store shelf indefinitely. It provides very few nutrients for the human body. But white flour can increase your weight. If you stop eating wheat and replace those calories with meat and vegetables, you will lose one to two pounds per week. In ten weeks, that is ten to twenty pounds—not bad for removing one unhealthy food.

2. Primarily drink water. Other than one to two cups of a caffeinated beverage, drink only water daily. God gave us water to replenish the fluids we lose. If you don't like plain water, add a slice of lemon and some stevia to it, or fresh berries, or drink carbonated, flavored water. There are many different recommendations for how much water you should drink per day. I follow this guideline because it takes into consideration your body size: drink half your body weight in ounces. For example, if you weigh 140 pounds, drink seventy ounces of water per day.

Keep track of your daily water intake and make sure you hydrate your body. Many times, we experience hunger when our body actually needs water. Next time you feel hungry, drink two glasses of water and see if your hunger subsides. If it has been less than three hours since you have eaten, most times the hunger will go away with water.

3. Take a daily probiotic. One of the easiest and best things we can do to improve our immune system is to take probiotics, as we discussed in the *Candida* section earlier. Buy a probiotic that contains at least ten strains of beneficial microorganisms. With each new purchase, try another brand with a different set of microbes. There are hundreds of probiotic strains, but we do not know which ones we need. That is why we should not take the same type of probiotic repeatedly.

Also, you can't get all your probiotics from a supplement, so consume one to two tablespoons of fermented products like sauerkraut or kimchi weekly (not yogurt, which doesn't provide enough benefits, or kombucha, which contains yeast and sugar). Dementia has been linked to a lack of gut microbiome diversity.[24] We must ensure our gut is healthy and contains the beneficial microorganisms it needs.

4. Limit your sugar intake. You should limit your sugar intake to less than ten grams of sugar per meal. The American Heart Association recommends limiting your calories from sugar. For most women that should be no more than twenty-five grams of sugar/day and thirty-six grams/day for men.[25] Be sure to check food labels to determine the number of grams of sugar per serving size.

5. Don't eat processed foods. Manufacturers create many prepackaged processed foods that are conveniently marketed in boxes and bags, and even portion sizes. Yet many of those foods do not contain any nutritional value, not to mention the extra cost you may pay for specialized packaging and marketing. The foods they are made from are stripped of their nutrients so they can sit on the grocery store shelf for months. If food does not go bad, it is not healthy. If a food spoils, it contains nutrients.

Food companies want you to buy more of their products so they will make more money. Therefore, they add sugar, salt, and other unhealthy ingredients to get you hooked. That's why "you can't eat just one." Outsmart the food industry and purchase fresh vegetables, fruits, nuts, seeds, and meat. Avoid the center aisles of the grocery store where the processed foods are shelved.

When you follow these five tips, you will be on your way to losing the excess weight you gained. Which one of these tips is easiest for you to implement? Start with that tip and move on to the next easiest one. Save the most challenging tip for last, after you have successfully created other healthy habits. You may also want to consider intermittent fasting.

Intermittent Fasting

Intermittent fasting occurs when you eat within a specific window of time. Scientific studies have proven that limiting food to specific hours is beneficial for the body and mind. I've been practicing it for years. I prefer a nine- to ten-hour window of eating. I eat dinner between six and seven p.m. and fast until the next morning around ten a.m.

Some people like to eat in an eight-hour window and fast the other sixteen hours, but that is too long a fasting period for me. Experiment with different time periods to see what suits you best. When the body is allowed to fast, or rest, from the digestion process, it is able to give energy to healing other systems.

Numerous studies show that intermittent fasting is beneficial. Check out these benefits:

- helps you lose weight, more specifically belly fat[26]
- reduces blood-sugar levels, which helps prevent or control type 2 diabetes[27]
- improves blood pressure and cholesterol levels[28]
- helps fight inflammation in the body[29]
- supports cell repair in areas of the body that need it[30]
- may protect against cancer and Alzheimer's disease[31]

These benefits will help us age gracefully and maintain our physical and mental capabilities. I recommend using intermittent fasting several days a week. I eat in this manner most of the time.

Here are some suggestions for attaining success with intermittent fasting.

- In the morning, drink two glasses of water upon waking.
- Go about your morning as usual, but do not eat breakfast.
- Stay busy, mentally and/or physically.
- Drink your usual caffeinated beverage.
- Every time you get hungry, drink another glass of water so you can delay eating breakfast as long as possible. I try to go until ten a.m., which works well for me.

- Ride out the hunger waves, which usually pass pretty quickly.
- Know the difference between needing and wanting to eat.
- Listen to your body. If you experience intense hunger, fatigue, or a headache—eat.
- When you eat, make sure the meal is low carbohydrate.
- Eat a healthy dinner that includes a wholesome protein source and loads of vegetables. You want to be satisfied but not stuffed. After dinner, don't eat anything.
- In the evening, try to keep your mind off food by watching a movie or reading a book.

You want to be satisfied and not hungry during the nine- to ten-hour eating window. Eating nutritious foods such as lean meats and vegetables is vital. Nutrient-rich foods keep your blood-sugar level steady and prevent nutritional deficiencies. Don't waste your calories on processed foods, refined carbohydrates, or desserts.

When you sit down to eat, pray and assess your plate. Does it resemble the food that comes out of the garden or off the ranch? If not, don't eat it. Food industries want us to consume more of their fabricated food items. I don't believe they care about our health. I think they are more concerned with their bottom line. Some people have suggested they get us hooked by adding sugar and salt to entice us to eat more.

It takes about a month of trying intermittent fasting to determine whether it is a good fit. If you are taking medication or under the care of a physician, consult with your doctor regarding this time-restricted eating practice. This is not for everyone, but I enjoy its benefits.

Intermittent fasting is an excellent weapon in the battle for weight loss, diabetes, and insulin resistance. Restricting calories may allow your pancreas to rest and heal.[32] To learn more about diabetes and insulin resistance, see chapter 6: Balance and Stabilize Your Hormones.

Imagine how you would look and feel after you shed your unwanted pounds. Say goodbye to those excess pounds and say hello to a healthier, younger-looking you. One of my secrets to fasting is staying hydrated because water fills me up, so I am not hungry for a longer period of time.

Stay Hydrated

God gave us water to drink, and it is vital to stay hydrated. If you do not consume an adequate amount of water, your body suffers. Some symptoms of dehydration include constipation, fatigue, dry skin and mouth, bladder and kidney problems, and high blood pressure because poorly hydrated blood is thicker. Our blood is 90 percent water.

Water nourishes and cleanses the body. The human body is comprised of 75 percent water, and we can't survive for more than a few days without it. While some people think drinking tea, coffee, or other caffeinated drinks will hydrate their body, they aren't doing the job as well as water can. In fact, caffeine is a diuretic, which, in large quantities, causes you to urinate more frequently and lose fluid.[33]

How much water should you consume? As I stated earlier, I believe your weight determines this. The guideline I use states that you should drink half your body weight of water in ounces. Pour the amount of water your body needs into a pitcher in the morning and drink it throughout the day. I drink at least a third of my daily water consumption before breakfast. Therefore, I am not hungry in the morning, and it is easy to fast until ten a.m. Don't drink any beverages after dinner to prevent getting up during the night to go to the bathroom.

PERSONAL AND PRACTICAL APPLICATION

1. Do you experience digestive issues such as bloating, belching, diarrhea, constipation, acid reflux, or stomach pain?
2. Have you ever had a stool test? If you've had any of these digestive issues, ask your medical professional about prescribing one for you.
3. Do you crave sugar, alcohol, wheat, and processed foods? *Candida* makes a person crave these types of foods. If you struggle with these symptoms, ask your medical professional to check for the presence of *Candida* in your digestive tract.

4. Do you have hard, thick toenails? This is a sign that candida may be infecting the nail bed.[34] Again, ask your medical professional about checking for this issue.
5. Do you suffer from a food allergy or an autoimmune disease? If yes, check for *Candida*.
6. Which weight-loss tip is easiest for you to implement? How can you begin to start making this change?
7. Have you ever tried intermittent fasting? When will you try it?
8. How much water should you consume per day? How do you plan to drink that much?

CHAPTER 3

THE SECRET TO STAYING PHYSICALLY ACTIVE

We do not stop exercising because we grow old.
We grow old because we stop exercising.
—Kenneth Cooper

One great fear many people face as they age is the possibility of losing their personal autonomy. We want to maintain independent lives and stay in our own homes well into our senior years. Long term, everyone I know wants to live long, healthy lives and die in a comfortable place surrounded by loved ones. Ensuring our bodies receive adequate physical exercise will help us succeed in that lifelong goal. Many aspects of aging prematurely (injury, osteoporosis, and chronic diseases) can be eliminated with lifestyle changes. The benefits of exercise are immeasurable:

- boosts energy, immunity, bone density, and mood
- improves sleep, weight loss, and mortality
- burns fat
- reduces stress, anxiety, blood pressure, falls, and hip fractures
- decreases chronic diseases such as diabetes, heart attack, stroke, hypertension, Alzheimer's, dementia, osteoporosis, arthritis, and depression

I believe God expects us to be stewards of our bodies. When you maintain an active lifestyle, you take care of the temple God gave you. You only have one body, and it needs to last a lifetime. You don't want your children or grandchildren to have to take care of you as you age. Being responsible for your body throughout your life will help prevent this. Ask God to give you the motivation to ensure your body receives adequate exercise.

Do you have active grandchildren you want to be involved with but need more energy and stamina? Do you want to enjoy your life and your family and all the years God gives you to the fullest? You need to be healthy, not simply for your sake but also for those you love and want to spend quality time with. Taking a walk with a loved one is an excellent way to spend time together, and it also keeps you on a healthy path to a longer life.

THE SECRET TO STAYING PHYSICALLY ACTIVE

If you already include regular exercise in your lifestyle, continue this habit throughout your life. When physical limitations require you to change your fitness routine, make adjustments but don't stop moving. The secret to staying active is to enjoy what you do. What type of activities did you enjoy as a youth? Did you play a sport or were you a member of the high school band? Pick up the instrument again and play beautiful music. Enjoy that time by allowing the right side of your brain to create. If you played ball, find a local team and join the sport. Joining a local team fosters camaraderie with others while enhancing physical fitness.

Sports were not for me. I am petite and couldn't seem to hit the softball into the outfield. The opposing team grabbed my grounders, and I was out before I ran to first base. Nor could I get that volleyball over the net. But I found other forms of exercise I liked.

Getting back to activities you enjoyed as a kid may motivate you to exercise more. Personally, I loved swimming as a child. My parents had seven kids. Every evening after Dad got home, he would take us to the clay pit—a small spring-fed pond. My brothers, sisters, and I jumped into the back of his truck, and Dad drove to his best friend's house who owned the pond. His best friend and kids jumped into the truck along with us, and we drove a block to their pond.

What an excellent form of entertainment for a slew of children. The dads got to talk and watch over us as we swam, while our mothers cooked the family dinners. We enjoyed playing with each other and got great exercise. Bedtime came easily for us.

My father taught us to swim when we were four. We had a bar of Ivory soap that floated, and at the end of our swim time, we would wash up in the pond using the soap. Exercise, friend time, and a bath all at once. It was the perfect solution for a big family. It saved water, and we didn't have to wrestle for the bathroom each evening.

Ever since I was a child, I dreamed of having a pool so I could swim anytime. When I dive into the water, it feels as if I have plunged into another world. Sounds are distorted; the water feels as smooth as silk; and my worries float away. I swim with goggles and a snorkel so I can stay under the water in my subterranean fantasy world.

Today, I have a pool in my backyard—dreams do come true. Swimming is a large part of my exercise regimen because I love it. In the late spring, I begin with swimming ten laps in my pool. The next time I swim, I increase my laps to eleven, and then twelve, and thirteen. After I've achieved twenty laps, I swim this many laps each time I swim. It takes about twenty minutes and provides a superior cardiovascular workout, as well as exercise for every muscle in the body. From May through September, I thoroughly enjoy swimming twice weekly.

During the winter months, I walk two miles a couple times a week. Walking strengthens bones and muscles and helps you maintain a healthy weight. Although running is an excellent cardiovascular workout, it wasn't right for me. It seemed to jolt the joints in my body. Human beings were meant to walk long distances. For centuries, we rode either horses or donkeys or used our feet. Only in the past hundred years have cars and planes become our primary modes of transportation. Jesus walked seventy plus miles from the Sea of Galilee to Jerusalem, and so did most Jewish men and their families for the Passover. Why is it so difficult for us to get out and walk a couple of miles?

I love God's nature. Walking through the woods calms my soul. I've created several walking trails in the woods on my five-acre property. Taking a break from writing to walk on the trails boosts my creativity.

Even if you live in an urban or suburban area, none of us is too far away from nature to find places for physical activity outdoors.

Planning hikes at cool destinations is fun and healthy. What better way to restore the peace in your heart, mind, and soul than walking in nature? When our family goes on vacation, we schedule several hikes to destinations such as waterfalls, lakes, or national parks. We exercise, bond, and view the spectacular world God created for us to enjoy.

Do you enjoy hiking in the woods? Next time you go, listen to birds chirp, feel the wind against your skin, smell the flowers, and feel the texture of a leaf. Spending time in nature restores the body through effortless attention—simply walking in the woods. God gave us nature to help regulate our emotions by calming our soul. God made the woods for us to enjoy, and it restores us physically and psychologically, which is amazing.

When we can't make it to a hiking spot, we can still be in nature by simply being outside. If you live in a place where there's more concrete than trees, you can still wonder and enjoy the sky, the sounds of birds, even smaller patches of grass or colorful potted plants in your neighborhood.

When the weather is bad, or I am talking on the phone, I walk around my house. It amazes me that after a forty-five-minute conversation with my daughter, I've walked two miles. I keep track of the miles via an app on my smartphone. I usually average one mile per day per month. That is not high, but it seems to be adequate for my body, along with working out at the gym weekly.

You may not enjoy being outside because God made us all different and each of us prefers various forms of exercise. Interestingly, the book *Eat Right 4 Your Type* theorizes that my Type AB-positive blood profile prefers less strenuous exercise such as swimming, walking, yoga, and dance.[1] That's probably why I did not relish sports, running, or step aerobics. We need to try different athletic endeavors to find what works best for our bodies and souls.

I like to dance. I don't dance much, but if I hear a great song, I may stop what I'm doing and dance. Many times, as I cooked dinner for my family, I listened to Christian praise music. It would not be uncommon for one of my daughters to walk by and see me lifting my arms, belting out the words, and worshiping God with all my heart while I danced

The Secret to Staying Physically Active

in the kitchen. Worship and dance release some powerful feel-good endorphins. Dance is a great form of cardiovascular exercise.

During the pandemic, as I listened to church services online, I danced around the living room during the worship sessions. At church, I usually sway back and forth with the rhythm of the music, but I don't dance. At home, I felt uninhibited and worshipped the Lord like David did in 2 Samuel 6:14. Each of us needs to find the exercise that works best for us.

Another form of exercise I enjoy is Christian yoga. I've been teaching a Scripture Yoga class at my church since 2004. I created two DVDs—*God's Mighty Angels* and *What the Bible Says about Prayer*—and two books—*Scripture Yoga* and *Yoga for Beginners*. Seniors love my class because it improves their flexibility. Some of my clients are in their eighties. If you desire a gentle form of exercise, yoga may do the trick. Check out my website at ChristianYoga.com.

Yoga has some amazing benefits:[2]

- enhances muscle strength and body flexibility
- reduces age-related gait or walking changes
- reduces stress, anxiety, and depression
- promotes and improves respiratory and cardiovascular function
- decreases blood pressure and cortisol levels
- improves sleep and balance
- increases serotonin levels
- reduces aches and pains
- manages and relieves chronic stress
- enhances overall well-being

These benefits help prevent falls. Seniors in my class say that yoga prevents their muscles and joints from being stiff, and they rarely miss a class. Through this form of exercise, muscles become well-defined, and the additional strength helps prevent injuries. The flexibility of the spine improves posture, which makes a person look younger. It also keeps the spinal disks supple. I have been doing yoga since my early twenties when I needed to decrease my stress as a student in a dual master's program. I believe performing yoga weekly has kept me younger-looking.

I tried step aerobics, but this form of exercise was not for me. I was not coordinated enough to get the steps right. I seemed to always lag behind the class members. However, it is great for coordination, muscle strength, and heart health. For years, I found excuses not to go to the gym—it's raining, I'm tired . . . you get the picture. Have you used those same excuses? When I became a yoga teacher at a gym, I had to show up. After my weekly class, I worked out. If at all possible, join a gym, the YMCA, or an exercise or yoga class where you have accountability. Some area churches have free or low-cost classes if a gym membership is not in your budget. Check around your area and in local papers to find a fitness class that matches your interests and budget.

When you work out with a group or join a team, you get to know the other participants, which provides both accountability and a social connection we need. God did not intend for us to live in solitude—but in groups who socialize. What type of group exercise activity could you join?

What about gardening? You may not think of this activity as physical fitness, but all that bending, squatting, and shoveling exercises many parts of the body. Housework can work out your body too. If you live in a northern climate, shoveling the snow is superior for fitness.

What activities do you enjoy? Even if you have some limitations, you can explore fun exercises such as water aerobics, chair yoga, Pilates, and stretching classes. Try different forms of activity until you find one you enjoy. Exercise must be fun to make it a routine. I dread running two miles in the Florida heat, but when I dive into cool, silky-smooth pool water, I enter my fantasy world that takes me away from all the troubles of this world. Now that is fun!

FALL PREVENTION AND EXERCISE ALTERNATIVES

As we age, we don't have the energy we had in our twenties. However, if we choose to give in to our waning energy and cease to exercise, our muscles atrophy and we lose strength. Plus, our bones lose density and break more easily. Accidents happen, but when we do not consistently take care of our bodies, we are more apt to fall. In fact, seniors are more prone to falling than at any other time in their lives. One fall could change a person's life.

A friend went through a six-month slump where he stopped exercising. With his inactivity, he gained twenty-five pounds, experienced hypertension, and lost muscle strength. This resulted in him falling off a ladder and hitting his head on a tile floor. When he awoke, he had no recollection of where he was or what he was doing. He suffered from a concussion, and the fall crushed two cervical vertebrae. The doctor told him he would most likely need surgery to fuse the vertebrae. One fall can lead to devastating results.

Exercise makes us stronger and more coordinated, so we are less likely to fall. Working out, attending yoga classes, and wearing supportive shoes help prevent falls. If someone who is functioning perfectly fine in their home in their eighties or nineties falls, this incident may cause them to suffer major life changes, such as having to live in an assisted living facility instead of returning to their home. Whatever we can do to prevent this from occurring, we should make it a priority. I've included fall-prevention tactics in the appendix.

If you are homebound, you can buy some hand weights and lift them twice a week or use exercise bands. Use three- to five-pound weights for lifting your arms at your side and in front of you. Use eight- to ten-pound weights for arm curls and raising the weights over your head. Lifting weights or exercising with bands is a great upper-body workout you can easily perform at home a couple of times a week, and you can do it sitting or standing.

You can also join an online exercise class. YouTube offers a variety of classes anyone can watch for free, or check your smart TV for such options that may come with it. If you have a sedentary work life, like me, get portable bicycle pedals to place in front of your chair. You can pedal away as you work. Now, that is an ingenious way to burn calories. Every time you take a bathroom break, do ten squats and lunges before plopping back down in your chair. Merely add a little movement during every bathroom break. Take a brief walk around the block when you go out to get the mail. Any type of physical movement gives you energy and clarity of mind.

AEROBIC EXERCISE AND STRENGTH TRAINING

We must commit to exercising our bodies four to six times per week. Ideally, four times should be aerobic exercise and two times strength training. Otherwise, our muscles deteriorate, bones lose density, and arteries clog. If we commit to exercising our body in this manner, we will feel more energetic and look years younger.

If you plan to begin a new exercise, check with your doctor to make sure you can perform specific activities. Be sure to start slow so you do not overdo it and injure yourself. You want to build your strength slowly. Begin and end any exercise routine with stretching. A good warm-up prevents injuries and decreases muscle soreness.

For aerobic exercise, choose a cardiovascular exercise, such as walking, biking, swimming, hiking, cross-country skiing, or using one of the following machines—treadmill, elliptical, rowing, stationary bike, or stair climber. You want to build up your endurance from twenty minutes to forty-five minutes of continued exercise. This includes your warm-up and cool-down stretches. Once you can perform forty-five minutes, it's time to vary your form of activity. So instead of always using the treadmill, try the stationary bicycle.

When performing aerobic training, you want to get your heart beating up to 60 percent of its maximum capacity. Determine your target heart rate by subtracting your age from 220 then multiplying that number by 60 percent. For example, a sixty-year-old would calculate 220 − 60 = 160, then 160 x 0.6 = 96. As a sixty-year-old, then, you want your heart to beat up to 96 beats per minute when exercising. If you don't want to take your pulse, download a heart rate app on your smartphone. You simply apply your finger to the camera lens. Or you could buy a pulse oximeter that includes the heart rate.

The simplest form of aerobic exercise is walking. God made our bodies to walk, and I believe this is one of the best forms of exercise we can perform. Jesus walked for four days from Galilee to Jerusalem. Lace up those excellent walking shoes, don a hat, and download a fitness app so it can record how many miles you walk. I use an iPhone, so the heart app automatically records my steps and mileage. You can also use your phone to play music, listen to an audiobook, or catch up on a podcast

The Secret to Staying Physically Active

as you go. If I'm walking over two miles, I put on my elastic knee band for more support.

For the first five minutes, start walking slowly to allow your body to adjust to movement. Then pick up the speed. Once you get into the rhythm of walking, your cardiovascular system pumps your blood through your arteries and capillaries. The pumping of blood benefits your heart and brain. After your walk, you will be more mentally alert and energetic. Depression and anxiety decrease with exercise, so it will improve your mental outlook as well. Strive for at least two miles per day at least four days per week.

My ninety-year-old mother-in-law (shown on the cover at age eighty-seven) walks over two miles every day. She takes no medication and lives alone. Walking is her secret to longevity without illness, disease, or a fall.

To entice myself to walk more, I started performing items on my to-do list while I walked. If you are an overachiever like me, you want to cross items off your list. So, grab your phone, lace up those walking shoes, and head out the door to make those administrative phone calls you've been putting off. You know, the ones where you have to call a company and be put on an extended hold. At least you can clock some steps while accomplishing those nuisance tasks.

Instead of sitting down with the Lord for your devotion time, go for a walk with him and pray. You could also listen to a sermon, podcast, or audiobook, or put on some music to keep yourself moving. Make it a game to see how much you can accomplish while walking.

If you have low bone density, use a weighted vest when walking.[3] This gives you more weight to carry during your walk, which builds stronger bones. Buy a vest that has the option to add more weight. Start with 4 percent of your body weight and work up to 10 percent.

If the weather permits, expose some skin without sunscreen to get vitamin D naturally through the sun. But protect your face by wearing a hat or sunscreen or both. Don't forget to apply a lip balm that includes a sun protection factor (SPF). At the end of your walk, slow your pace for the last two minutes to allow your body to adjust to an equilibrium state.

If you can't get outside to walk, walk from one end of your house to the other. Make it a habit to do this every time you're talking on the phone for an extended period. You will be amazed at how many steps you can take during a phone conversation. I always like to accomplish two things at one time, so I get more accomplished. Walking miles and catching up with a friend is a win-win.

If you have issues that prevent you from walking, buy a mini trampoline (rebounder). Jump up and down on the rebounder for a few minutes. Each day, add a couple of minutes until you can jump for fifteen minutes. Rebounding is another excellent form of aerobic exercise to get the blood pumping through your body and vital organs like the brain. It is gentler on the joints, too.[4] You could buy a rebounder that has a balance bar if you have issues with balance.

If you go to the gym, start your exercise routine by walking two miles on the treadmill. This prepares you for the rest of your workout by warming up your muscles, and it gets your blood pumping. If you prefer to use a stationary bike, stair-climbing machine, or elliptical, do that instead. Changing your form of aerobic exercise is an excellent way to work out different muscle groups.

After any form of aerobic exercise, be sure to hydrate. After my heart rate returns to normal and I stop sweating, I drink loads of water to replenish what was lost. Sweating releases toxins from the body. Be sure to get a shower to remove those toxins so they don't get reabsorbed back into your body. We will read more about how to eliminate toxins in chapter 5.

Strength training is also vital to maintain muscle strength, bone density, and prevent injuries. If we are sedentary, we lose muscle mass.[5] One of my visits to the doctor showed this on the InBody machine. I stepped on a scale and held onto the handles as the machine scanned my body to determine weight, muscle mass, and body mass index.

I had lost muscle. If I didn't start doing strength training more than one time per week, I would end up as a frail old lady. My daughters had been telling me this for a couple years. Why don't we listen to those closest to us who love us? The truth is hard to face.

If you've joined a gym, after your time on the treadmill, work out on the machines or use free weights. Now I work out with free weights at my home once a week and use the machines at the gym once weekly.

Working with a personal trainer is a great option to get you started with a strength training routine. I did this many years ago when I first joined a gym. Having someone take me through each machine helped me understand how to use it properly. Make sure you lift enough weight (but not so much that you injure yourself) and perform at least two sets of twelve to fifteen repetitions. You should allow your body two days to recover from concentrated strength training.[6] You could go more often if you work out your legs one day and your upper body the next. Strength training helps your body rebuild muscle tissue[7] to make you stronger and younger-looking. Well-defined muscles are visually pleasing.

You could also find a sport that strengthens muscles, such as bicycling, tennis, pickleball, kayaking, canoeing, swimming, and skiing. You can increase the strength of many muscle groups in a couple of months. If we are stronger, we can more easily perform daily tasks—taking out the trash, laundry, and cleaning. We need to understand that aerobics and strength training are key to maintaining our independence later in life. However, we can't be perfect, so increasing your activity level is an improvement.

FUN FAMILY FITNESS

Exercise can be a time of bonding with your spouse, grandchildren, and loved ones. Embracing an active lifestyle will go a long way toward your family adopting that same positive attitude. As you spend time with them while getting fit, you will knit your heart to your children, grandchildren, and spouse.

Exercise improves mood through releasing dopamine and serotonin in your brain. These neurohormones make you feel good and enhance bonding.[8] Walking with your partner can help you focus on each other without household distractions. Active time registers in a loved one's mind as love, and that love lasts.

Brainstorm with your family about enjoyable activities that incorporate physical fitness. Some ideas are bowling, swimming, canoeing, hiking, sports, and bicycling. Add to this list to personalize it for your family's interests. After your family brainstorms, plan when and how you will spend active time together. Get your calendar and plan when you will take a walk or go for a bike ride. This may include calling to schedule a canoe trip or a day trip for hiking. Playing and exercising with family will pay high dividends.

Whatever you do, make it fun and a regular habit for your family. Exercise is a blast, and it makes you feel alive. But it will not stick if you don't enjoy what you're doing, so make time for what you and your family will have fun doing on a regular basis. Try a variety of ideas. As you incorporate activities into your family's schedule, you draw closer together, and your relationships grow. Spending time as a family is vital, and there is no better way to do it than through fun, physically challenging activities. When you spend time with your kids and grandkids, you strengthen their self-image and help them become healthier. Together you are building a bond that will last a lifetime!

ADJUSTING TO LIFESTYLE MODIFICATIONS DUE TO INJURIES, AILMENTS, AND DISEASE

As we age, it becomes even more apparent that we need to take care of our bodies. After we sustain an injury or develop a disease, we must modify our lives to live with our limitations. We also need to brainstorm alternative health care practices that may improve our condition, such as massage, chiropractic adjustments, and physical therapy.

In my early twenties, I sustained injuries to my neck and temporomandibular joints (TMJ—jaw joint) from two car accidents. Before my first accident, a friend fixed my brakes but did not bleed the line of air. While driving home, I pumped the brakes repeatedly, but they did not work. I slammed into the car in front of me. I was not wearing a seat belt because before 1986 they were not required. That foolish mistake allowed my face to hit the steering wheel just below my nose. Blood gushed from a laceration to this area. The paramedics transported me via ambulance with sandbags on each side of my head in case I'd suffered spinal injuries. The emergency room performed X-rays and a scan of my jaw. I sustained a whiplash injury.

I suffered from TMJ dysfunction and had bilateral surgery to remove scar tissue and bits of cartilage. For nine months, I went for physical therapy treatments two to three times a week to treat my severe whiplash and back pain. Twenty minutes of ice packs followed exercises, massage, and electrical stimulation during each session.

Throughout my life since then, I've learned not to eat items that would require me to open my mouth wide—like a stacked hamburger—so as not to cause more pain. Have you needed to make adjustments in your life because of an injury, illness, or disease?

In my second car accident, I was wearing a seat belt. A huge truck slammed into me from behind as I was stopped because a car in front of me was turning left. From this second accident, I again suffered severe whiplash. The doctor ordered physical therapy for seven months. After the therapy ended, the doctor prescribed a TENS (transcutaneous electrical nerve stimulation) unit to wear to decrease my back pain. I attached the TENS unit electrode pads to the painful area of my back and neck to receive a low voltage electric current, which decreased pain. This treatment was much better than pain medication.

Needless to say, throughout my life, I've had to remain careful not to reinjure my upper back and neck. Since these accidents, I can't lift anything over fifteen to twenty pounds or my cervical vertebrae will rotate, which requires chiropractic adjustments.

I've visited my chiropractor every two to three months since these accidents. It seems like every time I overdo it with yard work or pick up something heavy, my back hurts. It is frustrating to not be able to do what I could before these accidents.

When I was in my teens, I would lift fifty-pound sacks of horse feed and pour them into storage containers. After the accidents, I couldn't do that. I've had to rely on others to help me or figure out ways to lessen the load and carry the item in two or three trips. I lost my full physical independence at a fairly young age, mid-twenties.

Many of us have experienced accidents or illnesses that left lasting limitations on our physical abilities. Yet this is not an excuse to stop exercising altogether. In fact, continuing the right kind of physical movement is even more important. We just need to work around these restrictions.

I didn't stop being active, but I did create my own rule for my body's limitations—don't lift anything over twenty pounds. Now that I am in my senior years, I've lowered that limit to fifteen pounds. I can't even pick up a heavy baby without my neck going out of alignment.

Still, at times we don't abide by our own boundaries. I've broken my twenty-pound rule many times in my life, especially with springtime yard work. I enjoy gardening and like to fertilize the yard and mulch the flower beds. When I lift bags of fertilizer or mulch, I reinjure my back and experience pain. My doctor prescribes muscle relaxers and physical therapy. It takes weeks to recover.

Massage therapy also helped my car accident injuries heal. A massage can seem like an extravagance, but when you relieve muscle tension and pain, you improve your life. How do your neck and shoulders feel? Are they tight? I've tried to schedule at least quarterly massage appointments to work on my neck, back, and the TMJ muscles. Massage is also an excellent way to release toxins that have been stored in your tissue. Always be sure to drink plenty of water after massage therapy so you expel those toxins.

My physical limitations have been frustrating and embarrassing to live with. "Sorry, I can't lift that item because it is too heavy, and it may hurt my back. I was in two car accidents when I was younger." I've repeated this statement so many times in my life and felt humiliated because of it. Have you felt humiliation because of your limitations? We need not feel this way because most of us have or will have to live within some sort of physical boundary at some point in life. The more we are able to admit this to others, and they to us, the more we can support and help one another.

What have you modified in your life because of an injury, illness, or disease? Life is full of injuries—physical, emotional, and spiritual. God helped me overcome those negative feelings of shame associated with my limitations. Just because I can't lift a baby does not make me less of a person. Our self-worth comes from God, not from being able to lift heavy items. Society's expectations of us are flawed, but God's expectations are not. Other than my family members and close friends, no one would know I have physical restrictions because I appear to look fine as I swim, walk, and teach Christian yoga. These physical activities I can do even with my limitations, and they keep me looking and feeling healthy.

ALTERNATIVE THERAPIES

In my thirties, I sustained a shoulder injury. As I held my horse with a lead rope, he got scared and bolted, which jerked my right arm.

Afterward I felt shoulder pain with certain movements. I adjusted and tried not to repeat that type of movement. I gave the injury months to heal. God created our bodies to heal, and often sprains and muscle tears can heal with time if they have not been severed completely.

After six months, I saw an orthopedic surgeon. She found nothing on an X-ray. An MRI was next. At my return visit, the doctor said that I did not have a rotator cuff tear, and she could do nothing for me but give me Voltaren gel for muscle pain. I went home and pondered what type of alternative therapy could improve my condition.

I tried weekly massages for a month, but the injury did not improve. The massage therapist recommended chiropractic treatment for my shoulder. My chiropractor had always treated my neck and back but not my shoulders or knees. At my next visit, he adjusted my shoulder, and it was healed. One chiropractic treatment was much less expensive than my whole workup with the orthopedic surgeon. *Why hadn't I thought of that before?*

In my forties, I did hours of yard work using a new-fangled tool I'd recently purchased to dig weeds out of my yard. I stuck the instrument into the ground above the root of the weed, pounded a pedal with my foot, and pulled up the instrument as it grabbed the weed by the root. It worked great; unfortunately, it worked a number on my hip. Have you ever pushed your body to its maximum capacity and sustained an injury? I did.

The next day my right hip hurt badly, as it did for weeks and then months. I could only bend down about ten times a day before pain seared through my hip. I felt defeated to be this young and unable to bend over and pick up my kids' toys.

Once again, I modified my life by limiting the number of times I bent down. I bought a grabber instrument that had a claw at the bottom of a three-foot rod. I pulled on a lever at the top of the rod to pick up my kids' clothes or toys.

My orthopedic surgeon ordered an MRI. There was a tear in my iliopsoas muscle and a cyst developed on the muscle tear. He gave me a cortisone injection, which relieved the pain. My family had their full-functioning mom back. But after eight months, the pain and limitations returned. I went back to the doctor, who gave me a second cortisone shot, which lasted for only a couple of months. Being a nurse, I knew that cortisone had negative side effects, so I didn't want a third shot. I chose to go to Mayo Clinic Jacksonville, where I used to work, for a full workup.

I saw the Mayo orthopedic surgeon and had another MRI. The next day, the doctor told me what I already knew, "You have a benign cyst on your iliopsoas muscle." He added something I did not want to hear. "I would not recommend surgery to remove the cyst because you may sustain more damage to the area from surgical scar tissue. There is nothing I can do to treat it. You need to learn to live with this limitation."

The doctor explained I was more physically active than most people and able to teach yoga and work out at the gym. My only limitation was that I could not bend down over ten times in a day without pain.

I had just spent a lot of money and three days away from my family at a premier medical institution to be told, "There is nothing that can be done to treat your condition." My hopes melted away. *I have to learn to live with this.*

Have you ever sought medical treatment hoping to relieve pain or symptoms only to find the doctor could not help or the treatment failed? Has a doctor said you need to learn to live with your limitations? It's frustrating, isn't it?

On my five-hour drive home from Mayo Clinic Jacksonville, I resolved to improve my mental outlook on my condition. I needed to change my attitude. Instead of focusing on what I couldn't do (bend down), I decided to focus on all the positive things I could do. The doctor was right, I could do a lot of other physical activities other than bending down. And my kids could pick up their own belongings.

I returned home to my family and used my grabber tool. I also began investigating alternative methods of therapy for my injury. We need to be our own health care advocates instead of only relying on traditional medical opinions. Alternative treatments used in conjunction with medical options give us a more holistic approach to our health.

I sought treatment with my chiropractor. He prescribed P-Wave (PiezoWave) therapy, which is a nonsurgical technology that uses sound pulses to treat acute and chronic muscle, ligament, and tendon injuries. I also tried deep-tissue massage. Still, I saw no improvement after either treatment.

My mother-in-law had recently bought an inversion table, which turns a person upside down. You get on the table, securely attach your feet, and slowly tilt the table backward so you hang upside down. Through inversion, the vertebral column and all joints hang freely without gravitational weight, which takes pressure off painful areas to help with healing. At first, you can only be inverted for five to ten seconds, but daily you increase that time until you get up to a minute. I used her inversion table and found some relief from my hip pain.

I bought my own inversion table and used it several times a day. After years of living with this injury and using this table, my injury resolved. Maybe the cyst finally dissipated. God programmed our bodies to heal themselves. Various therapies can heal our bodies. We just have to put on our thinking caps, investigate, and try them. We have to do our part to modify our lives and find alternative treatments to assist in the healing process.

We also need to stay physically fit in spite of limits. For instance, maybe you suffer from an ailment like plantar fasciitis, and it hurts to walk. However, you could get into a pool and swim with no pain. This is just one example of adjusting your activity based on your injury. We need to take care of those injuries at the time, and throughout our lives. We must learn how to adjust, modify, and accept our limitations without giving up on physical movement.

As you age, injuries may occur without an impactful incident. When I was in my fifties, I updated my home with new paint, door handles, and light fixtures. On the last day, I stored items in the top of a closet. I kneeled to pack the boxes and climbed a ladder to store them. The next day, my knee swelled like a balloon. The previous day, I had not felt an injury occur. These types of injuries come with age. I overdid it.

Now when I walk over two miles, my left knee hurts and sometimes swells, so I limit my walks to two miles or less unless I'm on vacation with my family and we walk more on hikes. At those times, I wear an elastic knee brace I bought at a pharmacy.

We can adjust our lives and figure out how to maintain an active lifestyle while modifying our activities for our injuries. It is sad how our body deteriorates as it ages. But that is the cycle of life. Each of us is born, and each of us dies. We must choose to modify where necessary but still maintain a healthy, physically active life as best we can for as long as possible.

PROPER FOOTWEAR

Last year, after returning from an active family hiking trip in Oregon, my massage therapist found knots in my calves. She told me I needed to change my walking shoes because I needed more arch support. Our feet are integral parts of our bodies. If your feet hurt, how can you be active? Invest in yourself and purchase supportive, therapeutic shoes. Cheap shoes can cause foot issues or promote falls. (Please see the appendix for fall-prevention interventions.)

Proper footwear helps prevent injuries and falls. Shop at a specialty shoe store where they can watch you walk and fit your feet with the best shoes for the type of activity you want to perform. I like to walk, not run, so I buy walking shoes. After you've had your shoes for a while, if you feel pain in your ankle, knee, or hip, it might be time to purchase another pair.

Foot bunions run in my family. I thought about having surgery to remove my bunions when I worked at Mayo Clinic Jacksonville. But my feet didn't hurt, so why would I mess with them just for attractiveness? I am petite with fairly small feet, but I need wide shoes. Small, wide shoes are hard to find. You have to shop in a large city or order shoes online. It takes work for me to find supportive shoes, but I do it because I invest in my body to prevent further injuries. I sure don't want any more.

As we age, our feet get bigger. Sagging arches and looser ligaments cause our feet to widen and our shoe size to increase.[9] If your old shoes are tight, this may be the reason. In my early fifties, my doctor told me to increase my shoe size.

It has been a journey for me to learn to live with my limitations. I lost my full independence in my twenties, but I am not less of a person because I have fewer abilities. I've turned to God and realized that my self-worth is from him and what he thinks of me, not what others think. As I've aged, it has been frustrating that small movements can injure me, and I can't be as busy because I have limited energy.

But even though these changes occurred, nothing is wrong with me. I've simply learned to adapt to the changes in my body. We all sustain injuries in our lives. We need to heal and adjust to our restrictions. Our limits do not make us less valuable.

BE INTENTIONAL

Have you used excuses to keep you from developing a healthy lifestyle with regular exercise? I did. I couldn't see how I could add a daily walk to my busy schedule until I learned how to walk and multitask simultaneously. Do you feel like you're too busy to exercise?

To improve, we must be intentional about fitness. Exercise does not have to be something you dread. Find something you enjoy that you can do long term, then plan how you will incorporate physical fitness into your life. Regular exercise prevents many chronic diseases, such as cardiovascular disease, diabetes, obesity, cancer, depression, hypertension, osteoporosis, and osteoarthritis. Physically active people have a lower risk of contracting these chronic diseases. It doesn't matter what exercise you do, as long as you do it.

PERSONAL AND PRACTICAL APPLICATION

1. The secret to having an active life is finding an exercise you enjoy and doing it regularly. What type of activities do you enjoy? How can you incorporate those exercise routines into your life?
2. How can you involve your family and/or friends in some of these activities?
3. Have you ever pushed your body to its maximum capacity and sustained an injury? What happened? How did you adjust?
4. Have you ever sought medical treatment hoping for pain or symptom relief only to find the doctor could not help or the treatment failed? How did that make you feel?

5. Have you been told to learn to live with your limitations? How did that make you feel? Did you find ways to adjust?
6. Have you investigated alternative treatments to assist in your body's healing process? What have you tried, and what were the results? What other options might you try if needed?
7. What have you modified in your life because of an injury, illness, or disease?
8. Have you felt humiliation because of your limitations? How can you overcome those negative feelings?
9. Have you figured how to adjust your type of exercise based upon your injury so you can maintain your physical fitness?
10. Have you invested in supportive, therapeutic shoes to help prevent falls and injuries?

CHAPTER 4

KEEP YOUR BRAIN YOUNG

When I look at the human brain, I'm still in awe of it.
—Ben Carson

Now that we have reviewed how to improve physical health, another component of overall well-being is brain health. With the rise of dementia and Alzheimer's in the past couple of decades, we want to do everything we can to preserve our mental acuity. First, we want to determine underlying causes and employ healthy-living habits to prevent or reverse symptoms of cognitive decline. This chapter reviews each potential contributing factor and a list of beneficial habits.

Dementia refers to a general term for the impaired ability to think, remember, or make decisions, all of which interfere with a person's life. This condition is uncommon under the age of sixty, but after that the risk increases.[1] However, dementia is not a normal part of the aging process.

Early treatment provides the opportunity to rule out other reasons for memory loss, such as stress, vitamin deficiencies, or medication side effects. Other causes of dementia-like symptoms are depression, thyroid problems, untreated sleep apnea, toxins, and excessive alcohol consumption. With treatment, the cognitive symptoms may be reversed. If someone is diagnosed with a specific form of dementia, it is important that they receive an accurate diagnosis, so they get the proper treatment and care. For example, dementia caused by a stroke would be treated differently than Alzheimer's, which is the most common type of dementia.[2]

My mother had a stroke when she was eighty-five years old, which caused dementia. However, she had no apparent symptoms of a stroke—no one-sided paralysis, slurred speech, or difficulty walking. But the stroke impaired her ability to make decisions. And one of those life-changing decisions was her refusal to get a dental cavity filled. Cognitive decline sneaks up on a person, and they lack the insight to understand that their mental abilities have been compromised.

About a month after the stroke, she visited me, but I did not know she'd had a stroke, nor did my sister who lived with her. I could see she had a cavity in one of her front incisors, so I took her to my dentist. When she was in the dental chair, she made an excuse to my dentist, "I would rather have my own dentist fill the cavity when I get home." I tried to talk her into getting it filled, but she politely refused. She seemed almost normal.

My sister scheduled a dental appointment right after Mom's visit. But our mother came up with a new excuse. Maybe she hated going to the dentist? The following month, her demeanor changed, and she became belligerent with unusual verbal outbursts. At that point, my sister knew something was wrong.

My four siblings and I worked together to figure out what was going on with our mother. My older sister flew to our mom's home and took her to the dentist. She had an abscessed tooth, and the dentist would not pull it until she had been on antibiotics for several weeks. After she completed the medication, my brother drove to my mom's and took her to the dentist for the extraction.

In the meantime, my younger sister, who lived with our mom, took her to the primary care physician who ordered blood tests and a CAT scan. Her vitamins D and B12 were low. Vitamin deficiencies can contribute to mental decline.[3] The doctor prescribed a large-dose vitamin D pill monthly, as well as weekly vitamin B12 shots. Getting mom to take the shots was difficult, as those with mild cognitive impairment (MCI) can be unreasonable.

My turn came next. I drove seven hours to take her to the doctor to receive the weekly B12 shots and a CAT scan. Have you ever dealt with someone who has dementia? It is like talking a two-year-old into going to the doctor for a shot. To our surprise, the CAT scan showed our mother had suffered a stroke several months earlier.

The stroke was the missing component of her health crisis. Mom's body functioned well, but her mind and decision-making processes had been impaired. This began the onset of vascular dementia, which lasted until she died at ninety-one. Vascular dementia is a common form of dementia that is caused by a reduced blood flow to the brain.[4] For my mother, it was from the stroke. Those caregiving years were tough. If you are a caregiver, you need to take care of yourself and not miss your own doctor or dental appointments.

While my mom was suffering from dementia, my father-in-law was diagnosed with Alzheimer's. This progressive brain disease affects an estimated 5.8 million Americans. It is the sixth leading cause of death among all adults and the fifth leading cause for those aged sixty-five or older.[5]

My father-in-law was genetically predisposed to this condition, as his mother was diagnosed with it in her early seventies. My "health nut" mother-in-law incorporated many of the modalities in this chapter, which held off his Alzheimer's until his mid-eighties—over a decade longer than his mother was diagnosed.

Alzheimer's disease develops because of multiple factors rather than one cause. The greatest factor is old age; the older you get, the higher your chances of getting it.[6] However, dementia is not a normal part of aging—this disease does not develop in every senior.

Alzheimer's disease destroys brain function, which leads to a mental decline (memory loss, language difficulty, poor decision-making) and behavioral issues (depression, delusions, agitation). With time, the person loses the ability to care for themselves. Most of us fear the loss of mental capabilities more than the loss of physical abilities.

The causes of dementia and Alzheimer's disease are multifaceted. They include a combination of environmental, genetic, and lifestyle factors such as toxins, pathogens, chronic inflammation, and the apolipoprotein E gene (APOE4). Cognitive decline can be prevented and improved by resolving the factors that contribute to it.[7]

However, a nonmodifiable factor is genetics. We receive two of each gene from our parents, one from our mother and the other from our father. If you carry one APOE4 gene, like I do, you have a 30 percent risk of getting Alzheimer's. If you have two copies of this gene, your lifetime risk is over 50 percent.[8] But there are lifestyle and environmental factors that can be employed to perhaps prevent the gene from "turning on."

Some people may not want to know their risk. But I did because now I understand how vital it is to carry out the suggestions in this chapter. Some people used to think that if you carried a gene, you would get the disease, but that is not the case. Even if you carry two APOE4 genes, you still have a 50 percent chance the gene will never activate, and you won't get the disease.

If you have a first-degree relative (parent, sibling) with Alzheimer's, you are also more likely to develop the disease. Diseases that run in families have more than just hereditary factors; they also share environmental and lifestyle upbringings and habits. But individuals can modify their unhealthy living habits and change their environment. Today's choices can preserve a healthy future.

TRAUMATIC BRAIN INJURIES

Unfortunately, a nonmodifiable risk factor associated with cognitive decline is brain injury. Traumatic brain injury (TBI) is a blow or jolt to the head or penetration of the skull by a foreign object. A mild TBI, characterized by a loss of consciousness or amnesia lasting thirty minutes or less, increases the risk of dementia. The more brain injuries sustained, the higher the risk of dementia. Repeated blows to the head through contact sports is associated with the development of dementia, so advise others to limit their children's contact sports.

SATURATED FAT

I have a family history of strokes. My maternal grandfather had several strokes in his seventies, my mother at age eighty-four, and a sister at age seventy-three. To decrease my chance of having a stroke, for example, I would need to decrease my consumption of animal products, which includes dairy and meat.[9] Fish and seafood are perfectly fine.

Dairy and meat contain saturated fat, which is the stuff that clogs arteries, including the arteries of the brain. Many of our animals are fed grain (glyphosate-containing corn) and live in unsanitary conditions, so they are given antibiotics to prevent infections. Some receive hormones so they can produce more milk or meat. Therefore, when we eat animal products that are not organic, we consume antibiotics, hormones, and glyphosate residue from their bodies.[10]

In addition, grain-fed meat is higher in omega-6, which is a type of unhealthy oil that we may consume too much of in the American diet.[11] The brain likes omega-3 oil that comes from olives, avocados, nuts, and seeds. To decrease our likelihood of a vascular stroke, especially if strokes and heart disease run in your family, it would be best to decrease your consumption of animal products.[12]

Consuming a diet with less saturated fat decreases cholesterol levels. And there are plenty of other foods that contain protein, such as nuts, seeds, quinoa, chia seed, avocados, lentils, beans, and much more. God gave us a wide variety of seafood and shellfish too.

INFLAMMATION

Chronic inflammation contributes to brain diseases.[13] Inflammation is the body's response to an internal problem. It's a normal reaction that signals the immune system to fight off an infection or heal an injury. Some visible examples of inflammation are a cut's redness and swelling or the swelling of a twisted ankle. Inflammation you can feel is when you run a fever with the flu or eat something bad and experience diarrhea.

God created the immune system to defend the body through a short-term inflammatory response. For example, the swelling decreases a week after the twisted ankle, or the diarrhea goes away after the bad food has been expelled. But when the body gets into a chronic state of inflammation, it leads to diseases such as diabetes, rheumatoid arthritis, heart disease, and dementia.[14]

You can determine if you have inflammation through a C-reactive protein blood test. It checks for inflammation in your body. If you have been diagnosed with dementia, you most likely have inflammation.[15] If you can figure out what is causing your body's chronic inflammation, you may be able to remove the root cause of it.

I always believe in getting to the root cause of a problem and resolving it versus masking the problem with medications. Increased intestinal permeability (leaky gut) is a common cause of inflammation. We addressed how to heal the gut in chapter 2.

High blood-sugar levels lead to chronic diseases, such as insulin resistance, type 2 diabetes, and dementia. Diabetes and prediabetes contribute to inflammation. Impaired glucose processing, a precursor to diabetes, increases the risk of dementia.[16] If you have type 2 diabetes, the condition can be improved through diet and exercise. Seek instruction from your doctor and follow the healthy eating guidelines provided in chapter 1.

In fact, some researchers suggest that dementia may be caused by what they call type 3 diabetes, or brain insulin resistance.[17] The solution is to lower sugar consumption.

Inflammatory foods we should avoid include:[18]

- sugar
- dairy
- fried foods
- grain-fed beef
- processed meat
- excessive alcohol
- high fructose corn syrup
- sugar-sweetened beverages
- refined carbohydrates (processed foods)
- partially hydrogenated oils or trans fats, such as margarine
- high omega-6 oils, such as corn, peanut, and sunflower oil
- gluten, if you are gluten sensitive
- any foods you may be sensitive to

Another dietary limitation that enhances brain health is to stop eating three hours before going to bed and fast for at least twelve hours between dinner and breakfast.[19] When you give your digestive system a break from eating, your body can use its energy to repair damaged cells from aging versus digesting food.

Natural repair of cell damage is an antiaging technique that God built into the body's systems. I believe we eat and drink so much that we hardly give our bodies the opportunity to repair cell damage because it is always digesting what we consume—it takes a lot of energy to break down food into the components the body uses—whereas, dietary restriction and fasting promote autophagy (see chapter 1).[20]

Try intermittent fasting several days a week, as we discussed in chapter 2. It will surprise you how easy it is not to eat in the morning. You can go for hours without eating and not even miss it, especially if you consume loads of water. If you feel hungry, drink two glasses of water. Sometimes I consume four glasses of water in the morning before I eat. That's half of my daily water consumption.

Chapter 1 reviewed which foods to eat and not eat. Eating a healthy diet provides many benefits, including weight loss, increased energy, improved mood, blood sugar stabilization, cognitive improvement, and decreased signs of aging. Healthy eating is fundamental to improving your overall health.

DENTAL HYGIENE

Another common cause of chronic inflammation is periodontitis or gingivitis, which is inflammation in the gums or around the teeth.[21] You wouldn't think dental hygiene had anything to do with brain health, but it does. Think of how close the mouth is to the brain. Consider how many germs the mouth contains, especially with periodontal gum disease. This type of disease is associated with dementia.[22] Therefore, I think we should optimize dental hygiene by using an electric toothbrush, dental floss, electric water flosser (Waterpik), and semiannual dental cleanings. These simple techniques may help prevent dementia.

PATHOGENS

Someone could have a chronic undiagnosed infection that contributes to cognitive decline. As we discussed in chapter 2, you want to make sure that your gastrointestinal tract does not harbor unwanted pathogens. Chronic urinary tract infections (UTI) definitely enhance a person's impaired mental status. My mother suffered from UTIs, and we never knew it until her mind declined further. We found D-mannose helped prevent these infections; it is a compound found in fruits. It is a great prophylaxis for recurrent UTIs.[23] Undiagnosed and untreated Lyme disease can play a role in dementia too.[24] Any of these infections would need to be treated by a doctor. Seeking medical attention early provides the best outcome, before more damage occurs.

PHYSICAL ACTIVITY

A fundamental component of brain health is exercise. Exercise improves brain function. Strive for thirty to sixty minutes, four to six times per week.[25] Yes, you heard me—four to six times per week. Aerobic exercise, where we get the heart beating faster, has positive effects on cognitive function. When the blood pumps faster through the blood system, it keeps the arterial lining of the arteries smooth, preventing buildup on the arterial walls.[26] I like to think of it as cleaning out a car's exhaust pipe when you hit the gas hard and fast. Regular exercise improves long-term memory and decreases the chance for dementia.[27]

VITAMIN LEVELS

When you get a physical exam, ask your doctor to check for vitamin deficiencies. I was on the low side of normal for vitamin D, and that made me feel tired. I finally got my level to the higher range of normal through taking a liquid vitamin D supplement instead of a pill. I also sit outside in the sun for twenty minutes without sunscreen several times a week. There is nothing like getting vitamin D the way God planned for us to receive it.

A symptom of low vitamin B12 includes mental problems, such as memory loss and behavioral changes. Vegetarians tend to have low levels of B12.[28] If you eat a diet with less meat and dairy, supplement with this vitamin.[29] I take a liquid B12 supplement that is placed under my tongue and tastes great.

Unfortunately, our foods do not contain the vitamins and minerals they used to, so taking a multivitamin is wise.[30] You want to ensure the following vitamin levels are normal:

- vitamin B12
- folate
- vitamins B1, B5, and B6
- vitamin C
- vitamin D
- vitamin E
- magnesium
- vitamin K2
- zinc

If any of these vitamin levels are low or on the low side of normal, take a supplement. Supplement recommendations were covered in chapter 1.

HORMONES

Just as your body needs appropriate levels of vitamins, it also needs adequate hormone levels. If a gland is not functioning properly and a hormone level is too high or low, this could affect your mental faculties. Your doctor can order blood tests to check your levels. We discuss hormones in depth in chapter 6.

TOXINS

Our exposure to toxins is higher today than ever before in the history of the human race.[31] We don't know what we've been exposed to, so a doctor would need to run tests to determine if we've had exposure to heavy metals, mold, or chemicals, like pesticides. These can be found through urine and blood testing. Toxins can play a role in the onset of dementia.[32] If they find high levels, you would need to detoxify. This subject is covered in chapter 5.

SLEEP APNEA

Sleep is integral to overall health, including brain health, and too little or disturbed sleep negatively affects our mental capacity. You should try to get at least seven hours of sleep per night.[33] Sleep apnea occurs when breathing repeatedly stops and restarts again while sleeping. Symptoms include loud snoring, gasping for air, and awakening with a dry mouth. When a person experiences sleep apnea, the oxygen level to their brain decreases. A pulse oximeter measures the oxygen saturation level. An optimal level is 96 percent and above.

A sleep study verifies if you have sleep apnea. An easier way to check your level is to purchase a pulse oximeter. In the middle of the night, before you get up to go to the bathroom, slip the oximeter on your finger and check the level. I did. My oxygen level was between ninety-seven and ninety-eight. A reading above 96 is normal. If it is not optimal, follow up with your health care provider. If you have sleep apnea, it needs to be treated to ensure your brain receives a sufficient amount of oxygen.

SOCIAL ISOLATION

Just as your muscles atrophy if you don't use them, so does your brain. Isolated, unstimulated lives do not provide the challenges a brain needs to grow. Strong social bonds, stimulating occupations, and purpose help decrease cognitive decline. More about the importance of community is covered in chapter 10.

COGNITIVE STIMULATION

Our brains continue to grow new neurons throughout our lives. There are many activities which stimulate this growth, such as playing games, solving crossword puzzles, putting together a physical puzzle, or learning a new language. Most jobs stimulate the mind in some manner. If you are retired, be sure to engage in some sort of cognitive activity for at least six hours per week.[34] TV does not count! I like to read, but someone else might like to listen to music. Keeping your mind active helps you to learn and prevents dementia. I recommend the app BrainHQ. It provides daily mind-stretching sessions that will help those neurons grow.

SUMMARY

Most people with MCI have at least one, if not several contributing factors. Addressing all the factors is critical to improve cognitive decline. Identifying the root causes of the decline and treating them will help decrease symptoms. To improve your chances of not suffering from cognitive decline, do the following:[35]

- Decrease inflammation.
- Exercise.
- Optimize vitamin and hormone levels.
- Determine and heal infections.
- Identify and remove toxins.
- Resolve sleep apnea.
- Perform socially and cognitively stimulating activities.

In the past, some people believed that once you got dementia, there was no reversing it. Now there is hope.[36] Besides resolving the root causes, you should also employ the following healthy habits, which help to decrease dementia risk factors:

- Eat a low-sugar, grain-free, anti-inflammatory diet with fewer animal products.
- Eat nothing three hours prior to going to bed and fast for twelve hours each night (from dinner until breakfast).
- Perform strength training and aerobic exercises several times per week. This is a fundamental component of brain health.
- Manage stress. Use stress reduction techniques.
- Optimize dental hygiene by using an electric toothbrush, electric water flosser (Waterpik), dental floss, and semiannual dental cleanings.
- Sleep eight hours each night. If you have insomnia and cannot sleep, take a supplement such as magnesium, melatonin, or tryptophan before bed.
- Engage with your family and friends—phone calls, lunch dates, walks.
- Perform cognitively stimulating activities.[37]

Factors such as your age and genes can't change, but other risk factors can be modified to reduce the risk of cognitive decline and dementia. The health of the heart and blood vessels affects brain health. A healthy heart ensures that the brain gets enough blood and oxygen pumped to it since the brain consumes 20 percent of the body's oxygen.[38] The healthy living factors discussed above protect the brain and heart.

I do not want to end up cognitively impaired with Alzheimer's like my father-in-law. His disease placed a terrible burden on his wife, who cared for him the last few years of his life until he died at his home. Nor do I want to suffer from a stroke like my mother and end up with dementia. The burden of my care would fall upon my three daughters, whom I love. I understand the devastating effects of watching my mother's brain and body waste away for years—until death finally ensued from dementia when she weighed less than eighty pounds. To decrease the likelihood of my APOE4 gene activating, I engage in the recommended healthy living habits. I hope you will choose to make lifestyle modifications to improve your brain health too. Your loved ones will appreciate your efforts.

PERSONAL AND PRACTICAL APPLICATION

1. Do you know someone who has dementia?
2. Are you a caregiver? If you are a caregiver, do you take time to take care of yourself? Do you need to schedule your own doctor or dental appointments?
3. Have you experienced a traumatic brain injury?
4. Are you eating too much sugar?
5. Do you have any of the contributing factors related to mild cognitive decline?
6. How could you try to resolve the root cause of a contributing factor?
7. What types of activities do you perform to stimulate your brain?
8. How often do you read a book? Do you have any books that you are interested in reading? Make a list and start reading.
9. Which healthy habits do you plan to adopt?

CHAPTER 5
ELIMINATE TOXINS: INSIDE AND OUT

Because no matter who we are or where we come from, we're all entitled to the basic human rights of clean air to breathe, clean water to drink, and healthy land to call home.
—attributed to Martin Luther King III

In the last fifty to one hundred years, our exposure to environmental toxins has escalated.[1] We don't often realize we live in a toxic world, where we are all exposed every day to poisonous substances that can harm the body. To live a longer, healthier life, we need to learn about the most common toxic substances, how to reduce our exposure to them, and how to detoxify from them.

A study published on March 17, 2021, in *Environmental Science and Technology* found 109 chemicals in the blood samples from pregnant women and their newborns.[2] These chemicals were from many different types of products, including forty used as plasticizers (phthalates), twenty-eight in cosmetics, twenty-five in consumer products, twenty-nine as pharmaceuticals, twenty-three as pesticides, three as flame retardants, and seven polyfluoroalkyl (PFAS) compounds used in carpeting, upholstery, and other applications. How did these substances get into their blood?

Have you ever thought about the chemicals and contaminants you are exposed to on a daily basis? Here's just one example from a recent trip I took with a friend. On our first day of vacation, I made coffee from the hotel room's small coffee maker. I placed the coffee packet in the flimsy plastic compartment. Hot water seeped through and dripped into a Styrofoam cup. Potential toxins included the coffee maker's plastic compartment and the Styrofoam cup. That's one example of how plasticizers can enter the body—we drink them.

Next, we went downstairs for breakfast. I got a cup of tea using a single-cup brewing machine. The tea dripped into a wax-lined paper cup. The plastic tea pod and wax-lined cup both contained possible toxins.

While driving to our destination, we stopped at a coffee shop for drinks again. My friend ordered a frozen cappuccino, and I got water in a plastic cup with a plastic straw. My friend applied lipstick before drinking her beverage. Likely toxins we ingested included her wax-lined cup, my plastic water cup and straw, and her lipstick. That was just in the first few hours of our day. Our bodies constantly absorb toxic substances without our being aware of it.

TOXINS

Contaminants enter the body in three ways—through the skin, lungs, and mouth. The skin absorbs chemicals from cosmetics, moisturizers, soaps, and sunscreen. We inhale air pollutants and flame-retardant chemicals from furniture. We eat and drink plastics, pesticides, and other chemicals added to our foods and beverages. These chemicals build up inside the body as we are exposed to them over time. Therefore, the longer we live, the higher our environmental toxicity level.

We should assess what we put on and in our bodies, just as we assess our food. Did God create it? Will the item harm or benefit the body? Anything toxic you put on or into your body must be eliminated in some manner.

Most of the chemicals we consume come from food. In chapter 1, we discussed chemicals used in growing food, such as herbicides and pesticides, but food manufacturers also add dyes, preservatives, and artificial flavors to many foods. Experts do not yet know if those substances are harmful or not.

The European Union has banned over 1,600 chemicals, but the United States has only banned nine of these.[3] So Americans are exposed to more toxic substances than people living in Europe.

The body can tolerate a certain amount of poison by detoxifying and excreting it through the liver, kidneys, skin, and lungs. Chemicals enter the bloodstream from the lungs, skin, or digestive tract and eventually reach the liver, which is our detoxification organ. The liver then converts the poisonous substance into a less toxic one that the body can eliminate through the bowels or kidneys. The kidneys filter contaminants out of the blood and excrete them in the urine. Sweating removes toxins through the skin.

The amount, type, and length of time you are exposed to a harmful substance will determine if your body can naturally remove it without adverse health effects. We come into contact with contaminants in our air, water, food, and many other products. If we want to live a longer, healthier life, we need to become more diligent at reducing the toxins entering our bodies and not rely on the body's detox system alone.

Air

We breathe air pollution from industry and transportation. Larger metropolitan cities contain higher levels of air pollution. If you live outside large cities, you are still at risk. For example, coal-burning power plants release mercury into the air.[4] I've known of lakes and rivers close to power plants that have contained fish with high levels of mercury. The authorities banned fishing from these bodies of water because of health reasons. The power plant close to me is on a river that flows into the bay. I wonder what the mercury does to the fish in the bay.

It seems impossible to change the air we breathe, but we can employ some interventions. To help mitigate the effects of air pollution, use a high-efficiency particulate air (HEPA) filter in your home because it removes up to 99 percent of dust, mold, bacteria, pollen, and other small airborne particles. I have a HEPA filter for each bedroom. The air circulates while I sleep and also provides excellent white noise, so no sound wakes me up. Since one of my daughters has severe allergies, I also have a whole house HEPA air conditioner.

If you use candles in your home, purchase those made from beeswax or soy instead of paraffin wax because paraffin emits benzene and toluene, which are neurotoxins.[5] I use an essential oil diffuser instead of candles. Each day I use an essential oil based upon how I feel and how the oil properties may improve my feelings. If I need energy, I use peppermint oil. If I need calmness, I use lavender oil. It is fun to match the oil with my mood to help improve it.

Mold is another potential household toxin when we breathe in mold spores. If you feel as though your home may have mold, purchase a mold detection kit and test for it. If mold exists, you may need to have remediation performed, which is a multistep process to remove the mold. To help prevent mold, keep the humidity level in your home lower than 60 percent and use a dehumidifier if needed.

Change your air conditioning filters regularly. After weeks or months of not opening the windows during long winters and summers, the air in a home gets stale. Open your windows and air out your house weekly. Spend time outside daily, if possible. Fresh clean air is best for breathing, in addition to the benefits of natural vitamin D from sunlight.

Water

Industrial pollution discharges harmful chemicals and compounds into the water supply. And now chemicals from prescription drugs and over-the-counter medications are getting into water systems. Tap water could contain metals, organic toxins, and traces of drugs. Do your part by not flushing unused drugs down the drain or toilet.

Public water contains unnatural chlorine and fluoride. Fluoride can decrease thyroid function, and chlorine can disturb your gut microbiome.[6] Try a water taste test by drinking water from the faucet versus filtered water. You can taste the chlorine in tap water. Chlorine is for the pool, not for human consumption.

Using a water filter will minimize your exposure to pollutants. A filter that has both reverse osmosis and a carbon filter are the superior options.[7] Check any potential filters for these two features. You can use a water filter in a pitcher (make sure the pitcher is glass and not plastic), under the kitchen sink, or in a whole-house system.

Eliminate Toxins: Inside and Out

Avoid single-use plastics such as plastic water bottles. This will help the environment and decrease your exposure to toxins.[8] If you must buy water for a trip, buy purified drinking water, distilled water, mineral water, or natural-spring water. Buy a stainless-steel-lined water bottle to refill. I have a twenty-four-ounce container, which also helps me keep track of how much water I consume daily. Three containers and I've drunk nine glasses of water. I try to drink one before breakfast, the second before lunch, and the third one in the afternoon.

Food

We ingest many of the toxins we are exposed to. While we covered healthy and unhealthy food options in chapter 1, our food choices are also about avoiding toxicity. We consume processed food made of engineered grains and oils that cause inflammation. Our produce contains residues from herbicides and pesticides that didn't even exist one hundred years ago. Pesticides are toxic chemicals that damage the liver, brain, and reproductive and nervous systems. Ingested pesticides tend to accumulate in the body's fat.[9] I believe that after they are stored there, the body does not allow you to lose that fat until the chemical is removed through detoxification. We will discuss how to detoxify later in this chapter.

Animals raised for meat are often fed grains with pesticidal and herbicidal residue. They are raised in overcrowded living conditions so they are given antibiotics to prevent infections. Some animals are dosed with hormones to promote rapid growth.[10] Meat from these grain-fed, antibiotic- and hormone-treated animals could promote inflammation and disrupt the gut microbiome in those who consume it.[11]

Anabolic hormones administered to dairy cattle contain endocrine-disrupting chemicals.[12] I believe that is why many young adolescents are entering puberty at a younger age. Buy organic dairy products instead.

The World Health Organization classified processed meats (hot dogs, ham, bacon, sausage, and some deli meats) as a group 1 carcinogen.[13] Most people have no idea that processed meats are right up there with tobacco, asbestos, and plutonium, which are listed as group 1 carcinogens. Also avoid prepackaged lunch meats. Buy meats at a deli, and make sure the attendant cuts slices from a hunk of meat that came from an animal versus meat that was shredded and formed into a mold.

Avoid canned foods and beverages to prevent exposure to the plastic substance used in the lining of most cans. Minimize your consumption of foods made with trans fat, preservatives, and dyes. Use storage containers made from glass to minimize the food's exposure to plastic.

Whenever possible, eat organic produce, free-range eggs, dairy products, and grass-fed meat. If you can't buy organic produce, choose the items with the least pesticide residue, such as those found on the Clean Fifteen annual list by the Environmental Working Group. We reviewed this list in chapter 1. Limit foods high in animal fat because many toxic substances build up in the fat of animals.[14] Examples of lean meats include skinless chicken, turkey, and fish. If you want to eat beef, choose leaner cuts such as round, chuck, sirloin, and tenderloin. Trim the fat from the meat before cooking.

You may not have control over the air you breathe, but you have control over the foods and beverages you consume. Choose to eat God's food as described in chapter 1.

Skin Care Products

The skin is your largest organ, and it absorbs what you put on it. Avoid cosmetics, skin care products, shampoos, and soaps that may contain toxins. Use a smartphone app (Think Dirty, Detox Me, EWG'S Healthy Living, Cosmethics, or Chemical Maze, to name a few) to scan the barcode of a product to determine its ingredients before purchasing. Minimize use of insect repellents and sunscreens. The Environmental Working Group has information about safe cosmetics, sunscreens, and insect repellants at EWG.org.

Heavy Metals

We are exposed to metals in unsuspecting ways. We come in contact with mercury through thermometers, coal-burning plants, and some fish. Arsenic is found in both pressure-treated wood and rice. Lead was used in old paint and outdated plumbing. We drink from aluminum cans and use antiperspirants containing it. Cadmium is in old batteries and cigarette smoke. These metals can accumulate in the soft tissues (fat) of the body.

Large predator fish contain more mercury because they live longer and eat small fish, thereby accumulating more mercury. These include tuna, swordfish, and bonita.[15] Limit consumption of these larger fish and choose small fish to eat instead, such as anchovies, cobia, cod, flounder, haddock, herring, mackerel, mullet, pollock, pompano, red snapper, salmon, sardines, sea bass, sole, tilapia, and whiting. Also, if possible, always choose wild-caught seafood over farmed. God's natural environment is much healthier than what humans create.

Dental amalgams (silver fillings) contain elemental mercury.[16] These fillings should be removed by a dentist who is trained to minimize exposure to the mercury during the removal.[17] I had my amalgams removed about a decade ago, but I did not realize I needed to have a specialist remove them. I had health issues around that time, and I still wonder if the mercury exposure contributed to them.

If your home was built before 1978, check for lead paint. Avoid buying products made with perfluorocarbon (PFC) that are used to make coatings—such as those found in nonstick cookware and stain-resistant coatings.[18] Buy stainless-steel cookware instead. Avoid using treated wood on decks or children's play structures because of the potential for arsenic leaching.

Plastics, Phthalates, and Paraben

Plastics are petrochemical products with hormone-disrupting chemicals that can harm pregnancy, neurodevelopment, and the immune system.[19] True plastic was patented in 1907. It began to be mass-produced after WWII.[20] Over the past sixty years, plastics have been introduced more and more into our food system and skin care products.

Bisphenol A (BPA) is found in plastics, canned-food linings, and thermal receipts. These receipts feel more slick than normal paper receipts. Unfortunately, BPA-free products may still contain Bisphenol S, which is toxic too.[21] A decade ago, I replaced all my plastic food storage containers with glass ones with plastic resealable lids. The lids usually do not come into contact with the leftovers. I do not freeze in plastic bags; instead, I use mason jars.[22]

Phthalates are a group of chemicals sometimes called plasticizers; they make plastic more durable. Phthalates from plastic bottles outgas (release a gas or vapor) and cause low testosterone rates.[23] Plasticizers are also found in skin care products and cosmetics like soap, shampoo, deodorant, perfume, hair spray, and nail polish. Phthalates are in plastic bags, plastic wrap, food packaging, vinyl flooring, detergent, and automotive plastics. Parabens, another hormone disruptor, are preservatives used in cosmetics, foods, beverages, and pharmaceuticals.

Europe banned several phthalates as well as five types of parabens, yet again, the United States has not done so.[24] Plastic wrap, bottles, and food containers can leach phthalates into food and beverages. Plastics, plasticizers, and parabens chemically mimic hormones, and therefore, disrupt them.[25]

Most people have plastic in their bodies as shown by the study published in *Environmental Science and Technology*.[26] These hormone-disrupting chemicals could be part of the gender identity crisis the United States is experiencing today. Baby pacifiers, bottles, and nipples are made from plastic. Think of the exposure our children receive from them.

Avoid eating foods stored or packaged with plastic. Do not use plastic containers for hot food or drinks because heat makes plastic release chemicals. Do not microwave in plastic; use glass or ceramic instead. Choose glass, stainless steel, or ceramic storage containers. I believe Tetra Pak containers are safe, as they are made of 75 percent cardboard.

Electromagnetic Frequencies (EMF)

Electromagnetic waves emitted by cell phones, tablets, Bluetooth devices, Wi-Fi routers, and other wireless communication devices are absorbed by the human body. Since these devices have only been mainstream for the past couple of decades, scientists are still studying the effects on our health. Studies in animals show that this type of radiation negatively effects the nervous system and brain function.[27]

Until we find out the long-term effects of EMFs, here a few tips to minimize exposure: increase your distance from the wireless device by three feet, avoid installing a smart meter in your home, and turn off the Wi-Fi at night. When talking on your smartphone use the speaker phone function instead of placing the device to your ear. Avoid wireless watches, sleep monitors, and headsets, as they emit EMFs.[28] Do not charge wireless devices by your bed or workspace. If you use a laptop, put something between your lap and the computer, such as a lap desk. If you give a child a wireless device to play with, turn it on airplane mode and switch Wi-Fi to off.[29]

STRATEGIES TO REDUCE TOXIN LEVELS

As you can see, we are exposed to more toxins than we imagined. To create a healthier home and lifestyle and lengthen your years, the following strategies can reduce your contact with them:[30]

- Don't wear shoes in the house. This reduces exposure to pesticides and lawn chemicals.
- Avoid using insecticides in your home. Use natural products instead.
- Replace reusable plastic food and beverage storage containers with glass or stainless-steel ones.
- Use natural cleaning products in your home. Most health food stores, and even some larger grocery stores, have these available, or you can make your own cleaning products using safe ingredients.
- Change or clean the furnace or air conditioning filters at least once every one to three months, depending on use.
- Use HEPA filters to clean the air in your home.
- Switch to natural brands of toiletries, including shampoo, toothpaste, antiperspirants, and cosmetics. Use nontoxic personal care products.
- Avoid using artificial air fresheners, dryer sheets, fabric softeners, or other synthetic fragrances, as they can pollute the air you breathe.[31]

- Avoid using lawn chemicals. Residue is easily tracked indoors where chemicals can persist in carpeting and on furnishings. Use natural lawn care methods.
- Test your tap water. If contaminants are found, install an appropriate water filter on all your faucets (even those in your shower or bath because the skin absorbs toxins).
- Select foam mattresses and furniture that are not flame retardant, as the retardant contains toxins.[32]
- Grow houseplants indoors to help absorb potentially harmful gases and clean the air.
- Ventilate your home—weekly when possible—by opening doors and windows on opposing sides of the room to facilitate air flow.
- Don't throw toxic substances down drains or toilets or in the garbage—such as gasoline, car oil, pesticides, paints, medicines, or solvents. Contact your local health department to find out how safely to dispose of those substances in your community.
- Sit in your car with the door closed when you pump gas, so you do not breathe the toxic fumes.
- Download a smartphone app to check every product for toxins before purchasing.

DETOXIFICATION

The body stores toxic substances in fat cells to protect the body.[33] The *total body burden* is a term used to describe the accumulation of toxic substances in the body. This level is affected by the amount of exposure and your body's ability to excrete the contaminant. These toxins can contribute to major health problems.[34]

Since we are exposed to more chemicals than ever before in history,[35] it is imperative that we detoxify on an ongoing basis. The liver, kidneys, and lungs remove poisons from the body. Often these organs are at their maximum capacity because we come into contact with so many different harmful products, many of which we are unaware of. Therefore, you need to periodically detoxify so your organs can work more efficiently.

Natural Detoxification Processes

It is imperative to have a well-functioning liver because it is the main detoxification organ. Eating more cruciferous vegetables (broccoli, cauliflower, brussels sprouts, cabbage, kale, bok choy, arugula, and collards) enhances the body's natural detoxification processes.[36] You can support your liver by taking the herb milk thistle, which is an ingredient included in many liver cleanse products.[37] To optimize the liver's cleansing ability, you could take one of these over-the-counter products: N-acetylcysteine or S-acetyl glutathione or liposomal glutathione.[38]

Our kidneys also help detoxify the body. If you have chronic kidney disease, minimize excessively salty foods and high phosphate-containing foods, such as processed cheese, so you don't overwork your kidneys.[39]

A therapeutic massage helps improve the lymphatic flow of toxic substances from your body. Make sure you specifically schedule a therapeutic massage. The day you receive a massage, be sure to drink loads of water before and after to help your body flush the toxins.[40] And soak in a hot tub with magnesium flakes (versus Epsom salt) to help your muscles recover.[41]

Dry brush your body with a body brush using slow circular motions. Start brushing the hands or feet and move toward your heart. The brushing stimulates your lymphatic system to release toxins, and it exfoliates your skin.[42] Once a week, I usually dry brush my skin before showering.

To enhance your body's detoxification capabilities, eat high-fiber foods from produce or take an organic psyllium husk supplement. The goal is to exceed thirty grams of fiber per day.[43]

Intermittent fasting, as discussed in chapter 2, promotes autophagy, which is the process where the body gets rid of old senescent cells. This process hinders cancer development and decreases inflammation.

In order to thrive and age well, given the environmental assault in today's polluted world, we need to go beyond the body's natural detoxification capabilities. You could ask your doctor to run tests to determine if you have toxic substances in your body. Or you could assume that you do and detoxify yourself through a general detoxification program. Health food stores carry numerous natural detoxification cleanses. Most toxins are stored in fat cells, so heavy sweating is an excellent God-given detoxification process.[44]

Infrared Sauna

Infrared saunas help remove toxic substances stored in fat cells through sweating. I believe many times people cannot lose fat until the toxins are removed. They try dieting and exercising but nothing works.[45]

Infrared saunas cause a person to sweat, which allows the removal of toxins through perspiration; in turn, regular sauna use has the potential to provide many beneficial health effects. Even heavy metals can be sweated out of the body during this detoxification process.[46] Be sure to shower with a nontoxic soap after using the sauna so you do not reabsorb the toxic substances you just expelled from your body.[47]

Fat cells are usually close to the skin. As the toxins are removed through perspiring, your skin becomes softer and clearer in appearance. And the red light of an infrared sauna promotes collagen formation, so your skin can become tighter. You might be able to lose cellulite too.[48]

You receive the best results if you use a sauna multiple times per week.[49] Some health gyms and spas contain saunas for their members. A local YMCA might as well. Check around in your area. A study published in *Journal of the American Medical Association* and *Harvard Health Review* showed a reduction in mortality with the increased frequency of sauna bathing.[50]

Infrared saunas heat up the body, which boosts your metabolism and helps you lose weight. Therefore, you burn more calories. The warmth may also boost the immune system.[51] And you may experience decreased pain. The sauna also decreases the risk of cardiovascular disease.[52]

We come into contact with thousands of chemicals that our grandparents never confronted. Your toxic load declines through eating pure organic foods, using chemical-free products, and removing stored toxins through sweating. Then your body can heal itself the way God intended.

Genetics and Epigenomics

Genes play a role in our health, but so do our lifestyles and exposure to environmental toxins. What we eat and how physically active we are can affect gene expression—basically, to turn on or off your genes. Epigenetics, a rapidly growing area of science, focuses on how our behaviors and environment affect the way our genes work.

Genes, which are composed of DNA (deoxyribonucleic acid) strands, determine our appearance and risk of having or developing genetic disorders. We receive our genes from our parents, and they received their genes from their parents. Therefore, diseases can run in families.

If your family has a history of certain diseases, you may have a gene variant for that illness. For example, my mother had one variant associated with macular degeneration. My genetic test showed that I have two variants associated with macular degeneration. One came from my mother and the second one from my father. My father's brother also suffered from macular degeneration in his eighties.

At birth, identical twins are the same genetically. However, over time, the epigenetic patterns of twins become different. These differences are thought to result from a combination of environmental influences that each individual experiences over a lifetime.[53]

Epigenomics (the study of epigenetic changes), thus, has become a vital part of efforts to better understand the human body and improve human health. Lifestyle and environmental factors (such as smoking, diet, and toxicity levels) may expose a person to pressures that prompt a chemical response leading to changes in gene expression.[54]

In this new scientific field, researchers are trying to understand the functions of genes. They are researching how chemical compounds attach or bind to DNA. When a chemical compound binds to DNA, it may cause certain genes to switch on or off.[55]

Not all epigenetic changes are permanent, as they can be added or removed in response to changes in behavior or environment.[56] For example, if a smoker quits, they can decrease their chance of activating a variant gene that causes cancer or a disease. Smoking increases my risk of macular degeneration genes turning on.[57]

I'm going to do everything possible to ensure my macular degeneration variant genes do not activate. I've seen an ophthalmologist who specializes in macular degeneration. He ordered baseline photographs of the back of my eye, so we know what the retina looks like with no disease. He recommended I take vitamin A, lutein, and zeaxanthin, as these compounds are found in the retina. My mother's genetic variant never turned on, and I hope mine never will either. Unfortunately, I have a sister who has shown signs of macular degeneration, so her gene has flipped the on switch.

Another familial disease in my family is breast cancer. My maternal grandmother died of breast cancer in her early forties. Genetic testing was not available in the 1940s, but we are fortunate it is today. My mother is the only daughter out of three who did not carry the BRCA1 variant. Both of her sisters had breast cancer. One of their granddaughters also had breast cancer in her forties. With genetic testing, she found out she carried the BRCA1 variant. This variant increases the likelihood that you will develop breast cancer from 13 percent to 72 percent.[58] Prostate cancer is also associated with this gene.[59]

My cousin with breast cancer has two daughters. One of them carries the BRCA1 gene, but she is on a regimen to help prevent the disease and receives early detection testing. Since she is in her twenties, she has an annual MRI of her breasts and a doctor's manual exam to check for cancer. Mammograms are not recommended until she is in her thirties.

Early detection improves our treatment outcomes. Since genetics is a rapidly growing scientific study, each of us should check with our doctor, high-risk breast cancer specialist, and genetic counselor regarding the latest recommendations.

If you know a specific disease runs in your family, you can have genetic testing to determine if you have that gene. If you do, you can employ preventive measures to try to prevent the gene from turning on. We used to think that once you had the gene, that was it—you would get the disease at some point in your life. Today, we know that is not true because lifestyle and toxic exposure have an integral effect on whether or not the gene activates.[60]

We can't change our genes. But we can alter the expression of them. We can turn off or on a gene by our lifestyle choices and detoxification.[61] Scientists are working to more clearly understand the epigenomic changes that can lead to cancer and other genetic-related diseases. For instance, understanding all the changes that turn a normal cell into a cancer cell will speed efforts to develop new and better ways of diagnosing, treating, and preventing cancer and genetic-related diseases. Improving your lifestyle is an extensive project, so take it on in bite-sized chunks.

PERSONAL AND PRACTICAL APPLICATION

1. Have you ever thought about the chemicals and contaminants you are exposed to on a daily basis? Make a list over the course of one day to get an idea of how many toxins you may not have noticed before.
2. Do you ever think about whether an item you eat, put on your skin, or breathe will harm or benefit your body? How can you become more aware of each product or food your body is exposed to? How can you educate yourself more about such toxins?
3. Were you aware that you should never flush unused drugs down the drain or toilet? Take an inventory of any expired medications you may have in your home and dispose of them correctly.
4. How many dental amalgams (silver fillings) do you have? Schedule a conversation with a dental professional at your next visit to discuss their removal.
5. Do you drink from plastic water bottles? Do you store leftovers in plastic containers? What changes will you make now for you and your family to decrease this exposure from toxins in plastics?
6. Did you know that skin care products may contain toxic substances? Take the time to find the right app for you to

monitor toxins in your personal-care items. Check this chapter for suggestions of apps and lists that will help you.
7. Have you tried to lose fat, but it wouldn't budge no matter what you tried? I believe that you need to expel the toxins from the fat first, before you can lose the fat. How does this information give you hope for more positive changes in your weight?
8. Do you have access to an infrared sauna? If not, research where you might locate a place to visit and find out their prices and possible discounts for monthly membership.
9. Are you surprised to find that variant genes can turn on or off? Does this give you more hope if you know you have a predisposition to a gene-related disease? If you have diseases in your family, I encourage you to talk to your doctor about the appropriate genetic testing.

CHAPTER 6

BALANCE AND STABILIZE YOUR HORMONES

I believe that the greatest gift you can give your family and the world is a healthy you.

—Joyce Meyer

As we have seen, toxicity is a major contributor, both environmentally and personally, to how we age. A more specific danger of toxins is how they disrupt our hormones. A faster loss of hormones accelerates aging,[1] yet we can help alleviate this effect and keep our hormones in balance with a healthy diet and exercise.[2]

Hormones affect our mood, libido, metabolism, and how we deal with stress.[3] When hormones are not balanced, it decreases the quality of one's life. Many of our hormones are part of human physiology, though some are gender-specific. Likely the most familiar of those is estrogen because of the way it impacts a woman's body when it begins to decrease.

Menopause officially begins when a woman has gone twelve months without having a period. Most women experience menopause by age fifty-one. However, symptoms of decreasing hormone levels begin many years before menopause. This early period is called perimenopause.[4] Unwanted symptoms can accompany the onset of menopause for years.

Despite the difficult symptoms, menopause brings some benefits. We no longer experience menstruation or need to be concerned about getting pregnant. This can be a wonderful time to finally not have to use birth control. Usually, by this time, couples experience an empty nest too, so these years can be a delightful time of romance revival.

If you are single, be aware that sexually transmitted infections are elevating in the senior population.[5] Personally, I believe in following God's rules by not engaging in sexual activity outside the bounds of marriage. But for those who do, protection is crucial to prevent getting a sexually transmitted disease.

If you are sexually active, be sure to schedule an annual pap smear to ensure you do not have cervical cancer. Ninety-nine percent of cervical cancer is caused by a human papillomavirus, which is transmitted sexually.[6] Over eleven thousand women in the US are diagnosed with cervical cancer and about four thousand women die from it annually.[7]

Part of the aging process includes a natural reduction in hormones. This is the way God designed our bodies. Going through menopause is like experiencing puberty again. During puberty, our hormones raged as they increased, and our bodies developed into a woman or a man. Again, the body undergoes a tempest as our hormones decrease with age. Unfortunately, our muscle mass, libido, and overall well-being plummets as well. All these changes prepare our mortal bodies to ultimately die. However, we can help our hormone levels decrease more gradually and maintain more youthful vitality for a longer period.

HORMONES

Before we can learn how to manage our hormones, we need to understand more about what they are. Hormones are chemicals our organs and glands release to help the body function properly. When one of these organs does not work right, this hormone disturbance causes disease and illness, and may affect other organs.[8] Some organs and glands, along with their accompanying hormones, are as follows:

- ovaries—estrogen and progesterone
- testicles—testosterone
- adrenal glands—cortisol and adrenaline
- thyroid—thyroid hormones
- pancreas—insulin

Both men and women experience declining hormones as they age. For men, it is generally gradual over decades. But for women, this decline is more rapid over a few years before and after menopause. Both men and women may experience unwanted symptoms from declining levels.

Menopause

Some women don't experience menopausal symptoms, but I haven't met any who haven't. As women enter perimenopause, their ovaries make less estrogen.[9]

When ovaries produce less, adrenal glands create androgens, which can convert to female hormones and reduce menopausal symptoms.[10] Unfortunately, in our high-stress society, many women experience adrenal fatigue, so the adrenals do not keep up with the body's needed demand.

Menopausal symptoms make women miserable. Some common symptoms include the following:[11]

- irritability
- hot flashes
- excessive sweating
- sleep disturbances
- mood changes
- vaginal dryness
- sexual issues
- bladder problems
- physical and mental exhaustion

During this transitional stage of life, women are at a higher risk of depression, anxiety, and mood changes.[12] All the changes occurring in the body can overlap with mental health symptoms. I know it did for me. If you were naturally calm and logical prior to menopause and now you are not, it is probably this life change and not your mental status. Stressful life circumstances exacerbate these symptoms. Having an open discussion with family members, as well as your doctor, can help.

Natural remedies can decrease unwanted symptoms. Relaxation, yoga, and counseling help manage stress and depression. Exercise, along with limiting caffeine and alcohol, improves sleep. Lubricants help with dryness so you can enjoy sex again. If you experience pain with sexual intercourse, your doctor can prescribe estrogen cream to administer vaginally. The estrogen will revitalize this area of your body.

Urinary tract infections (UTIs) may increase after menopause too.[13] My mother was prone to suffer from UTIs and so was I. D-mannose helped me prevent these infections. This supplement is a compound found in fruits. It is a great prophylaxis for recurrent UTIs. I take one 500 mg capsule about twice a week, and it's been years since I've experienced a UTI.

My Menopausal Story

In my late forties, I began noticing perimenopausal symptoms. I was more uptight and irritable—no longer patient and understanding with my children and husband. I couldn't handle stress like I used to. Little things really got to me, and I would blow up. I thought to myself, *I am not who I used to be. Who is this woman?*

I didn't like myself, and I can see how my family didn't either. I started experiencing hot flashes. The intensity of the heat within me seared throughout my body. I would open the refrigerator door and stand there to cool myself down.

In the middle of the night, I would awaken and be up for hours. The insomnia was dreadful and miserable. Nothing I tried made me fall back to sleep. In the early hours of the morning, I finally would find sleep, but then the alarm would ring. I would start the day exhausted. No wonder I was so irritable and short-tempered.

I noticed my hair was greasy no matter how much I washed it. I quit using conditioner, but that didn't help.

My husband knew of a compounding pharmacy that provided counseling. They recommended a local gynecologist who specialized in bioidentical hormone replacement. I set up my appointment. The physician ordered saliva testing. Besides my plummeting progesterone, I was also experiencing adrenal fatigue. To alleviate these issues, the doctor prescribed adrenal fatigue vitamins and progesterone cream that the pharmacy compounded for me.

The two primary sex hormones for females are estrogen and progesterone. The doctor said I had too much estrogen and not enough progesterone, which is called estrogen dominance.

Progesterone is like a purring kitten, but estrogen is like a feral cat. No wonder my calm self turned into a raging woman who could easily lose control. I had to get more of that purring kitten back.

Before bed, I would apply the progesterone cream to four areas of my body, alternately. These areas included the soft, pale skin under my upper arms, breasts, inner thighs, and each side of the groin. I kept a calendar of where I applied the cream each day so I could rotate the application.

The progesterone worked. After a month or so, I could finally sleep. The oiliness of my hair went away. But most importantly, I regained my patience and self-control. I was kind again and responded to my family and stress appropriately. For me, the bioidentical hormone was a lifesaver.

I kept taking bioidentical hormones for several years after menopause. In my mid-fifties, I stopped. Instead, I bought a natural, plant-based progesterone cream from a health food store. I used it once or twice a week if I experienced a hot flash. I believe slowing the reduction of progesterone helped me age gracefully.

If you are in your forties and suffering from irritability; weight gain; thinning, oily hair; and an inability to manage stress like you used to, I highly recommend you see a doctor to measure your hormone levels. Your physician may prescribe bioidentical hormones. You do not want to take a synthetic hormone replacement. Once your doctor balances your hormones, you and your family will notice the positive changes in you.

Find a doctor who specializes in bioidentical hormone therapy because not all doctors do. Bioidentical hormones should be prescribed individually either through a cream or orally. Using bioidentical hormones will increase the quality of your life in your senior years.

Osteoporosis and Bone Density

Our bone cells, like all our body's cells, are constantly regenerating throughout our lifetime. Osteoporosis occurs when new bone creation does not keep up with bone loss. The likelihood of increased bone loss for both men and women increases with age as hormones decline; so does the risk of falls and fractures. Low bone density and muscle strength, along with poor balance, increase the risk of falls too.[14]

(There's a reason why after a certain age, every medical questionnaire or interview asks if you've fallen lately!) Improving your bone health can decrease your fall risk.[15] Seek to minimize the consequence of any fall late in life, as it can be a life changer. Check out the appendix Fall Prevention for more tips to avoid falling.

With menopause comes the increased risk for osteoporosis.[16] Ask your physician to test your bone density. If the results show your bones are getting weaker, ensure you are getting enough vitamin D and perform weight-bearing exercises.

Lifting weights actually causes our body to create more bone, which increases the density in the bones bearing the most weight.[17] Join a gym or use weights at home to ensure your bones don't become osteoporotic.

Urinary Incontinence

As we age, urinary incontinence increases.[18] But we can take action to prevent it. In nursing school, I learned about the pelvic floor exercise called Kegels. This is when you squeeze your bottom as if you were trying to stop the flow of urine.

You can find out how weak your muscles are in this area by trying to stop the flow of urine when you are on the toilet. Most of us have weak muscles down there because we do not exercise them. Add these techniques to your workout routine a few times a week to prevent urinary incontinence and strengthen these muscles.[19] These exercises can be done standing or sitting, but standing is more effective:

- Squeeze your pelvic floor for ten seconds, then relax. Repeat this for two sets of fifteen repetitions.
- Pretend your pelvic floor is an elevator. Shut the elevator door and move the elevator to the first floor, and then the second, and finally the third floor. Hold for ten seconds. Now move the elevator down to the second floor, then the first floor, and open the elevator door and relax. Repeat this three to five times.
- Squeeze your pelvic floor and then immediately relax. Perform two sets of fifteen repetitions.

After a couple months of exercising, try to stop your flow of urine again. You'll be amazed how much more control you gain over this part of your body through exercise. It may even improve your sex life!

God designed man and woman to unite to become one physically. Sex is a delightful experience God gave us to enjoy with our spouse. If it wasn't so enjoyable, there wouldn't be so many babies in the world. I hope you have found sex to be a pleasurable, desired experience with your partner. If not, talk with your spouse and physician about the possible reasons. Help is available through foreplay, lubrication, estrogen cream, and a mutual understanding between lovers. A desire to please the other person is an immense part of satisfying intimacy.

Men and Testosterone

Testosterone is the primary male hormone. In men, testosterone is primarily produced in the testicles, and with age, their function decreases. Testosterone affects the healthy function of organs and tissues throughout the body. Testosterone levels naturally decline with age, usually beginning in the forties. Lowered testosterone levels can decrease libido and muscle strength.[20]

A deficiency of testosterone is common in elderly men.[21] Some common symptoms of lowered testosterone in men include the following:[22]

- lowered mood and depression
- reduced muscle mass and strength
- decreased energy
- low sperm count
- decreased libido
- reduced sexual function

No man wants to be impotent. Therefore, he should ask his doctor to check his hormone levels. Testosterone replacement therapy has been found helpful in older men's sexual function, bone density, and mood.[23]

Doctors can prescribe testosterone gels that are applied like progesterone cream to sensitive skin areas. Testosterone patches are also available.

Other factors besides aging can affect testosterone. Lower levels are more common in men who are obese or have type 2 diabetes and obstructive sleep apnea.[24] A healthy diet and exercise routine help decrease these risk factors. Ultimately, positive lifestyle habits will improve low testosterone. Many men do not address the symptoms associated with low testosterone, but if those symptoms interfere with their quality of life, they should discuss symptoms and options for treatment with a physician.

Adrenal Fatigue

The adrenal glands are located above each kidney. They secrete two primary hormones, adrenaline and cortisol, which help you respond to stress—often called the fight-or-flight response. Chronic stress can cause the adrenals to get stuck on overdrive because they cannot keep up with the body's need for these hormones. Since the body is designed to produce these hormones during times of stress, not continuously, we may exhaust our adrenal glands over a period of time if we do not reduce stress. When the adrenals can longer make sufficient amounts of stress hormones, the condition is known as adrenal fatigue.[25]

You've used up too much of your flight-or-fight adrenal stress hormones. Another factor is the adrenal glands become the primary source of women's sex hormones after menopause, which can reduce the body's adrenal abilities.[26] Some symptoms of adrenal fatigue include:[27]

- low energy levels
- problems with sleep
- impaired immune function
- depressed mood
- changes in behavior and emotional regulation
- craving salt or sugar

Now those glands are worn out and so are you. You have to rely on caffeine to get you through the day. When I suffered from adrenal fatigue, my biggest symptom was utter exhaustion. I did not want to get out of bed. I barely had enough energy to walk one hundred feet to my barn to feed my horses.

As usual, diet and lifestyle can play a factor. These lifestyle conditions contribute to adrenal fatigue:[28]

Balance and Stabilize Your Hormones

- poor diet with lots of junk food
- high caffeine
- skipping meals or excessive dieting
- lack of sleep and exercise
- low vitamin D[29]
- overexercising
- toxins

Stress is not the only factor that wears down our adrenal function. Our bodies were not meant to come into contact with so many stressful situations. Overactive adrenal glands can accelerate aging.[30]

Elevated cortisol levels also cause your body to store more fat around the belly and the sides of your face. From photographs, I can see my face was rounder and puffier when I was experiencing adrenal overdrive. Excessive cortisol also stimulates your appetite for sugary, high-caloric, fatty foods.[31] Here comes the inner tube around the belly. Being overweight, especially around the waist, can contribute to insulin resistance and type 2 diabetes. An overproduction of cortisol can also lead to depression and anxiety disorders.[32] What a nightmare. And you don't even realize what is going on in your body.

The good news is that adrenal fatigue can be reversed. First, you need to be tested to see if you have adrenal fatigue. My doctor diagnosed me with a saliva test. If you suspect adrenal fatigue, consult an experienced physician in the field of testing and treatment for this diagnosis, as not all are proficient in this field.

To overcome the overuse of these essential glands, you need to decrease your stress. The next chapter, Overcome the Battle with Stress, teaches my prescribed stress-reduction techniques. Besides reducing stress, these natural hacks may help restore the adrenal glands:

- Get out in the sun early in the morning for twenty minutes.
- Don't wake up before it is light outside.
- Sleep until nine a.m. as many mornings as you can.
- Eat about an hour after you wake up or before ten a.m.
- Eat nutritious snacks between meals so your blood sugar does not drop.
- Don't overexercise or skip meals.
- Decrease sugar and caffeine consumption.

- Combine a protein-rich food with a fruit so your blood sugar does not spike.
- Drink an adequate amount of water.
- Chew thoroughly and take digestive enzymes with meals.
- Evaluate your schedule to minimize duties.
- Rest during the day.
- Laugh.
- Take magnesium if you crave chocolate.
- Take vitamins E and C.
- Take ginseng.
- Try acupuncture.
- Sprinkle food with kelp.
- Instead of sitting, lie down to watch television or read.
- Drink licorice root tea.[33]

I discovered many of these techniques from *Adrenal Fatigue: The 21st Century Stress Syndrome*. I employed most of these tips and put them together as a cohesive list of natural hacks.

My doctor also prescribed adrenal vitamins. At first, I had to take them five times a day. But as I incorporated these strategies listed above, plus my stress-reduction techniques in chapter 7, my adrenal glands healed. The healing process was slow, but with time and patience, my body recovered in about a year. It can take months or even a year or two for your adrenals to recover. So don't give up. Keep working to restore these vital worn-out organs.

I tend to slump into adrenal fatigue when I experience long periods of chronic stress (like during a recent home renovation due to water damage). When I recognized my slump, I started taking my adrenal vitamins, decreased my caffeine, and rested when my body needed a break. God created our glorious bodies in his image. We can heal them if we understand the issue within them.

Thyroid Function

The body's hormonal system is interrelated. No one hormone operates on its own; each affects the other. For instance, when your adrenal glands rev up into overdrive and produce too much cortisol, this can cause issues with your thyroid gland.[34] The thyroid is a small gland at the base of the neck, near your larynx or Adam's apple. The thyroid is the engine for your metabolism. When your thyroid doesn't work properly, everything in your body slows down. Your intestinal system slows, causing constipation, and your metabolism slows, so you gain weight.[35] Some common symptoms of an underactive thyroid or hypothyroidism are as follows:[36]

- weight gain
- constipation
- fatigue
- sensitivity to cold
- dry skin
- slower movements and thoughts
- muscle weakness and aches
- thinning hair
- a puffy face
- memory issues

Hypothyroidism occurs when the thyroid gland does not make enough thyroid hormone. Usually, the symptoms begin gradually so you do not notice them. You may think your fatigue, added weight, and memory problems are a normal part of getting older. But they are not.

The adrenal glands rely on the thyroid to function correctly and vice versa, so when one gland goes out of whack, it affects the other.[37] If you experience symptoms of low thyroid function, make an appointment with your physician to get your thyroid checked. When an ear, nose, and throat doctor performed a physical exam of my thyroid, he thought he felt nodules. An ultrasound revealed five small non-cancerous thyroid nodules. My doctor and I monitor them regularly to ensure they do not become cancerous.

When you have blood tests and your levels come back at the lower 10 percent of normal—the level may not be in the most optimal range for your well-being. I never understood why my doctor told me my thyroid levels were normal when my bloodwork showed my thyroid function in the very low range of normal. If my level increased by 50 percent, I would feel better.

If you only have a few symptoms of hypothyroidism or your levels are on the low side of normal like mine were, you can treat your low thyroid function naturally. I did. To promote a healthy thyroid, be sure your multivitamin includes B, C, and A vitamins, selenium, and zinc. Ensure you eat foods with good sources of iodine (eggs, fish, and seafood) or use salt with added iodine. My favorite snack is organic, heirloom popcorn that I pop on the stove. I top it with coconut oil, iodized salt, sea kelp, and dulse. These sea vegetables are high in iodine, so I benefit my thyroid while enjoying my snack.

If you are diagnosed with hypothyroidism, your physician should try to determine why because more than one disease process (adrenal overdrive) can lead to hypothyroidism. Most doctors will order a thyroid antibodies test to determine if your condition is caused by Hashimoto's disease, which is the most common cause of hypothyroidism and affects 2 percent of the population in the United States.[38]

Hashimoto's disease or Hashimoto's thyroiditis is an autoimmune disorder where your body's antibodies have gone rogue and attacked your thyroid instead of a foreign substance. This condition is most common among middle-aged women. With conventional medicine, the primary treatment is thyroid hormone replacement. However, this treatment does not solve the reason the condition exists. I always believe in trying to resolve the root cause so the body can heal naturally—the way God intended it to.

An autoimmune disease occurs when the immune system makes antibodies to protect the body from foreign substances, but mistakenly attacks the thyroid or other body parts. Some potential root causes of Hashimoto's include leaky gut syndrome, food allergies and sensitivities, nutritional deficiencies, and other autoimmune diseases. A diagnosis of one autoimmune disease increases your likelihood of getting another. Autoimmune disease causes are multifactorial, including genetics, diet, stress, and environmental influences.[39]

In chapter 2, Keep Your Gut Healthy, I explained leaky gut syndrome and how this condition can lead to an overactive autoimmune response. To heal your thyroid, determine which immune-reacting foods you have consumed, and stop eating them. These include gluten, grain, dairy, sugar, and soy.[40] Begin to eliminate them from your diet, as well as fast foods and processed foods. All of these contribute to an unhealthy gut and can make you vulnerable to autoimmune issues.

You may wonder, "What can I eat?" Remember, in chapter 1, Eat to Live Longer, we discovered the best foods to eat—God's vegetables, fruits, meat, nuts, and seeds. Additionally, you may need to eliminate all grains. Take the steps in chapters 1 and 2 to change your diet and heal your gut.

In addition to healing your leaky gut, decrease your toxic exposure, especially to hormone disruptive substances as we learned in chapter 5, Eliminate Toxins: Inside and Out. Find a physician who treats the root cause of Hashimoto's thyroiditis. A friend of mine found the right doctor, and in six months, she lost fifty pounds, and her thyroid began working again. Her transformation was miraculous.

Insulin Resistance and Diabetes

The pancreas secretes the hormone insulin. When a person eats or drinks something high in sugar or carbohydrates, the pancreas releases insulin to decrease the blood sugar. If your body continues to be bombarded with too much sugar, your pancreas can wear out, like your adrenals, or your body may become insulin resistant. Insulin resistance makes your cells unresponsive to the insulin your pancreas releases to bring balance. As a result, your pancreas has to produce more insulin (like your adrenal glands going into hyperdrive).[41]

Unfortunately, the United States is on the verge of a type 2 diabetes epidemic, because about 10 percent of Americans have diabetes and 90 percent of them have type 2 diabetes.[42] And 38 percent of the adult population is prediabetic, as of 2019.[43] The percentage of people with type 2 diabetes increases with age as well. Risk factors for this disease include the following:[44]

- being obese or overweight
- physical inactivity
- smoking
- being age forty-five or older
- having close relative with diabetes
- having high blood pressure

With these risk factors and the continued consumption of high-sugar and high-carbohydrate foods, a person may become a type 2 diabetic. Think of your pancreas as an organ with a limited amount of insulin. If you continue to eat high-sugar and high-carbohydrate substances, you use up all your insulin. When your insulin runs out, you become diabetic, so you have to get your source of insulin from medication. It is a life-threatening condition when it remains untreated.

On the other hand, type 1 diabetes, also known as juvenile diabetes, is an autoimmune disease where the body attacks the pancreas. This results in a deficiency of insulin. Type 1 diabetes is different from type 2. You can't change your genes, but many of the type 2 diabetes risk factors are lifestyle choices—eating, weight, physical activity, and smoking. With every bite of unhealthy foods, you move closer to running out of insulin (diabetes) or wearing out your pancreas (insulin resistance).

Insulin resistance is enhanced when a person has too much visceral fat around their abdomen. Studies have shown that belly fat makes hormones and other substances that contribute to inflammation in the body.[45]

A person is prediabetic when their blood glucose levels are higher than normal. My sister was prediabetic, but within three months she reversed the condition through changes in her diet and activity. In the US, one out of three people are prediabetic and many do not realize it because prediabetics usually do not experience symptoms.[46] Some common symptoms of diabetes are listed below:[47]

- thirst
- hunger
- frequent urination
- blurry vision
- fatigue
- sores that heal slowly
- weight loss
- tingling or numb hands and feet
- dry skin
- more infections than usual

Type 2 diabetes takes several years to develop, so the symptoms gradually increase.[48] However, some people do not experience symptoms. If you suspect you are prediabetic or diabetic, see your physician so he or she can order simple blood tests to determine a diagnosis.

A person with prediabetes has up to a 50 percent chance of developing diabetes over the next five years.[49] But you can do something about it. Change your diet and increase your physical activity. One of my readers told me that his diabetic condition reversed when he implemented the steps in my book *7 Steps to Get Off Sugar and Carbohydrates*.

If you have diabetes, you need to be diligent to care for yourself, including the following:

- Monitor daily blood sugar tests.
- Take medications as prescribed by your physician.
- Eat a low-carb, low-sugar diet.
- Exercise.
- Perform diligent foot care.
- Visit your doctor regularly.

Complications of diabetes can lead to kidney disease, slow-healing sores, nerve damage (neuropathy), and vision problems. Diabetes is the leading cause of new cases of adult blindness.[50] Be sure to get your vision checked. Since wounds heal slowly, and neuropathy causes numbness of the feet, be sure to wear shoes or slippers while at home. Check your feet for sores. If you have one, be diligent to care for the wound. A friend of mine just had his foot and ankle amputated because of diabetic complications. To help prevent these complications, manage your blood sugar and blood pressure, eat a healthy diet, and exercise.

God created our amazing bodies to be healthy all our lives. Our hormones are interactive and work with each other. When we do not take care of our bodies, the organs and glands that produce hormones can wear out and stop working, which causes disease. If we can catch any health issues early, we can reverse the negative effects and maintain a healthy body as we age.

Treat your body with the respect it deserves, as God intended. When you care for it, your body will take you further on a healthy and satisfying ride of life.

PERSONAL AND PRACTICAL APPLICATION

1. Have you experienced symptoms of menopause? Did you ever consider using bioidentical hormones? When will you schedule time with your gynecologist to discuss hormone testing and treatment?
2. Have you had a bone density test? If not, schedule one at your next doctor's visit. Have you broken any bones in the past few years? How can you reduce your risk of this happening again, or for the first time?
3. Do you exercise using weights to help build your bone density? If you don't, when will you seek out a gym or purchase some weights to use at home? Be sure you meet with a trained fitness instructor or find a guide to show you how to use weights correctly so you don't harm yourself.
4. Do you suffer from urinary incontinence when you sneeze or cough? If yes, when can you add Kegels to your exercise routine?
5. Have you suffered from symptoms of adrenal fatigue? If yes, what lifestyle techniques mentioned in this chapter will you incorporate to improve your adrenal health?
6. Do you feel as though your aging has accelerated? What do you think is the cause?
7. Has your doctor ever checked your thyroid function through a blood test or physical exam? Do you experience any symptoms of an underactive thyroid?
8. Are any of your blood tests on the low side of normal? If yes, which ones? What can do you to improve those levels?
9. Do you have some risk factors for diabetes? If yes, what changes can you make to improve your chances of not acquiring this disease? If you've already been diagnosed, what lifestyle changes will decrease your risk of complications now and in the future?
10. How important is it to you to age well? What tips from these first six chapters do you want to incorporate into your daily living to ensure greater health and longevity?

CHAPTER 7

OVERCOME THE BATTLE WITH STRESS

Being in control of your life and having realistic expectations about your day-to-day challenges are the keys to stress management, which is perhaps the most important ingredient to living a happy, healthy, and rewarding life.

—Marilu Henner

We can be proactive about the aging process in many facets of our health, like food, exercise, and decreasing toxins. Still, a silent, unseen killer lurks in the shadows—stress.

While we don't see stress, we definitely feel it. We encounter stressful situations daily. It's hard to keep up with today's changing technology and fast-paced world, which adds to the ongoing pressure in life from finances, work-life balance, family, and the future. We feel the effects of stress in tense and aching muscles, hypertension, irritability, or worry. Stress accelerates aging, makes you sick, and shortens your life span. Therefore, it is vital to figure out how to alleviate it. What do you do to lessen your pressure? Do you go to the gym, walk in nature, or snack on comfort foods?

Stress causes many of us to eat more than we should and to crave carbohydrates, sugary comfort foods, and junk food. These processed foods provide a quick rush, which is what we seek, but then cause the blood sugar to crash, which makes us feel rotten. This mood change from blood-sugar fluctuation can in turn cause anxiety.[1] If we understand the connection between stressful emotions and eating habits, we can be proactive by having satisfying, nutritious snacks on hand.

We can also fight our love handles, and love of sugar, by calling on God to give us peace. God's peace is not like the world's. His peace is not temporary. His peace is a true antidote to debilitating stress.

PHYSICAL EFFECTS OF STRESS

Everyone experiences pressure, but how our body reacts to it is what can harm us. Stress is the body's reaction to real or perceived harmful situations. When you feel threatened, a fight-or-flight response occurs that affects many of the body's systems. Short-term stress raises the heart rate, breathing, blood pressure, muscle tension, and glucose levels as the stress hormones—adrenaline and cortisol—release from the adrenal glands.[2] Your body is ready to defend itself. Once the crisis resolves, the body systems return to normal.

When stressed muscles in the neck tense up, this can lead to headaches and migraines. For some, the strain affects the digestive system with pain, nausea, and bloating, or more trips to the bathroom. Contrary to popular belief, stress does not increase acid production in the stomach nor cause ulcers. The harmful gut bacterium, H. pylori, that we discussed in chapter 2, usually causes ulcers.[3]

When under pressure, individuals may eat much more or less than usual. Or they may turn to tobacco, alcohol, or drugs—anything to relieve the pressure they feel. These vices can lead to addiction. More pain to deal with.

We are all different, and some people may handle stress better than others. Maybe they didn't sustain as much trauma in their life as others did, so they have better ways to cope with daily stress. What causes tension in one person may not affect another the same way. In small doses, stress can help us accomplish tasks. Yet God designed our bodies to handle stress and the fight-or-flight response in small doses, not on an ongoing basis or at constant high levels.

We have two nervous systems in our bodies: the sympathetic (fight-or-flight) and parasympathetic (rest/digest).[4] Many people have such high-paced lives that their bodies get stuck in the sympathetic mode. When a person is chronically stressed, it is hard to turn off the physiological response. The body moves into overdrive. Chronic stress over a long period drains our strength and energy because the nervous system continues to trigger the secretion of cortisol and epinephrine. When strain becomes chronic (long-term), it can have devastating health effects.[5]

Ongoing stress increases the risk of high blood pressure, heart attack, and stroke, in addition to metabolic disorders such as diabetes and obesity. Chronic stress compromises mental health as well and can cause depression, irritability, and moodiness. Long-term elevated levels of cortisol can lead to chronic fatigue and adrenal fatigue.[6] This takes months, if not years, to recover from.

Most of us are so used to being uptight that we don't recognize the physiological symptoms of it. Some mental and emotional symptoms of stress include the following:[7]

- depression, loneliness, anxiety
- moodiness, irritability, agitation
- feelings of being overwhelmed
- racing thoughts
- worry
- nervous behaviors such as nail-biting, fidgeting, and pacing
- feeling disorganized, unfocused, forgetful
- procrastination
- impaired judgement
- feeling pessimistic, negative
- feeling worthless, low self-esteem
- increased use of alcohol, tobacco, or drugs

Physical symptoms of stress include the following:[8]

- headaches
- digestive issues such as nausea, diarrhea, or constipation
- appetite changes
- muscle tension and pain
- racing heart, chest pain
- low energy
- jaw clenching and teeth grinding
- shaking or sweaty hands

- insomnia
- decreased sex drive
- increased colds and infections

Stress can initiate or worsen health problems, such as these below:[9]

- cardiovascular diseases, such as high blood pressure, heart arrhythmias, strokes, and heart attacks
- gastrointestinal issues, such as acid reflux, irritable bowel syndrome, and colitis
- mental health disorders and anxiety
- obesity and other eating disorders

Ultimately, you want to relieve your tension through positive mechanisms so your body can return to its normal state. Through stress-relieving techniques you can obtain your body's equilibrium, increase energy, and keep stress from contributing to a shorter life.

STRESS MANAGEMENT

The first step in controlling stress is understanding the symptoms associated with it. From the previous list, which symptoms do you suffer from? Take a moment to assess how stress affects you physically so you can acknowledge its effects and begin to fight against it.

The second step in managing stress is understanding what causes it. Is it your job, mother-in-law, or neighbor? Create a list of the things that cause you pressure. Next, figure out which stressors you can change and begin to modify your life to accommodate those changes.

When I experienced adrenal fatigue, I made a list of both the beneficial and stressful elements in my life. I had to figure out what caused my stress and manage it because my body was so depleted that I could barely get out of bed. My doctor put me on three adrenal fatigue vitamins five times a day—that's fifteen vitamins per day!

My beneficial list of items included gardening, attending Bible study and yoga, reading, walking, napping, and working out at the gym. My harmful list included cooking dinner, arguing with my husband, driving my three daughters to their activities, skipping breakfast, drinking soft drinks, going grocery shopping with the kids, talking with my aunt on the phone, and disciplining the children.

Next, I figured out what I could easily change—I began eating healthy breakfasts and stopped drinking soft drinks. Then I solicited help for managing other items. I had my kids cook dinner once or twice a week and asked my husband to handle grocery shopping or watch the kids while I went on my own. I had to find ways to manage my stress and allow my body to heal. It took over a year to get my energy back and recover. God made our bodies to heal. Mine finally did.

I also had to proactively incorporate the list of beneficial items into my daily life. I needed to eat well and exercise. I also loved to read, walk, and attend Bible study, so I made sure to create those positive habits in my life.

As for my aunt, whose phone calls nearly always made me stress unnecessarily, I used my caller ID, so if I didn't have the time or energy to handle a long conversation, I would not answer her call. I also practiced valid reasons to get off the phone, such as to prepare dinner or help one of my kids with homework.

In my current job, I've chosen not to answer emails first thing in the morning. Someone else's crisis should not take over my day. To decrease my strain, I've chosen to answer emails from three to five p.m. That way I do not give the most energetic part of my day to others. Instead, I get items on my to-do list done before I answer emails.

Time blocking is another excellent mechanism to manage daily stress. Block out a period of time to perform a task (gardening, work project, and so on). Turn off the phone and work on that project for the block of time allotted. After you've completed the task, you will feel satisfied for getting it accomplished, not stressed because it's still on your mind.

What alleviates pressure is unique to you. Determine how to manage your stress and anxiety. My body responds well to doing yoga, exercise, and getting a massage. Therefore, I teach a Christian yoga class weekly and work out at the gym afterward. I also schedule a monthly massage. My body deserves to be taken care of properly. These techniques lessen my body's fight-or-flight response. Learn how you can make stress relievers a priority in your life, depending on what will bring your body the best results.

The third step to managing stress is learning when your body is going into the stress response. When I suffered from adrenal fatigue, I figured this out and can still recognize it today. It's usually when I am running late—like when trying to leave to teach yoga. I get in a hurry and become clumsy as my body tenses up because I am trying to do things quickly. I recognize what is happening, so I purposefully tell myself, *Susan, you are not in a hurry. Calm down. Breathe. No one is dying; it's okay.* Through this recognition of what is happening, I can stop my body's automatic reaction to the pressure.

By being more self-aware, you can also recognize when your body initiates the fight-or-flight response. Figure out when this occurs and talk to yourself to calm down. Most times it is perceived stress versus a real-life crisis.

In summary, the steps to manage stress include the following:

1. Understand your symptoms associated with stress.
2. Determine what causes your stress. List the items and figure out how to manage them better.
3. Notice when your body goes into the fight-or-flight response and talk yourself down, so you do not respond to the strain.

These steps will help reduce the effect of stress on our bodies. Yet for some of us, additional harmful stressors have become a pattern in our lives. In particular, many people are bound by a habit of worry, increasing our anxiety levels on a constant basis. Therefore, we need to focus on how to stop worrying and obtain God's supernatural peace.

WORRY

Jesus teaches us about worry in Matthew 6:25–27: "That is why I tell you not to worry about everyday life—whether you have enough food and drink, or enough clothes to wear. Look at the birds. They don't plant or harvest or store food in barns, for your heavenly Father feeds them. And aren't you far more valuable to him than they are? Can all your worries add a single moment to your life?"

Through this passage, Jesus tells us not to worry and to instead trust that he will take care of us. But not worrying and trusting are hard to do when your Social Security check is a fraction of what you lived off of before you retired. It's hard not to worry when you are waiting for your doctor's appointment to see if the biopsy is cancerous. How in the world do we stop our minds from racing through all the negative potential outcomes?

Jesus gives us the solution in Matthew 6:34: "So don't worry about tomorrow, for tomorrow will bring its own worries. Today's trouble is enough for today." The key is to focus on today and only deal with the burdens of the present. We shouldn't think about the issues we have to deal with tomorrow or next week—only today.

When I was getting my divorce, I couldn't think about the outcome. If I did, I would go crazy. I did not know how my three children would react and whether they would take sides. Would I lose my daughters? Fear consumed me. I cried out to God, and he gave me Matthew 6:34 as my theme verse for that year. Every time fear crept into my mind about my future, I recited the verse out loud. I chose to only think about each day, one day at a time.

Another truth Jesus taught in Matthew 6:27 is that worry cannot add a single moment to your life; instead, it can actually shorten your life. Chronic stress harms the body. But we can manage our anxiety and take control of our life.

GOD'S PEACE

Obtaining God's peace seems elusive. Jesus told us his peace was different from the world's peace. What did he mean and how can we find his divine peace? The secret comes from 1 Peter 5:7: "Cast all your anxiety on him because he cares for you." In this verse, cast means to hurl or throw, like you would cast a fishing line. We need to hurl away our fear to God and replace it with his peace.

We can hand any situation to God and ask him to intervene. Pray for God's intervention to be done in his timing. Then you take the burden off yourself and place it into God's capable hands. Giving God our burdens is a choice—keep them or cast them to the Lord. What burden do you need to cast to the Lord?

In Matthew 11:29–30, Jesus explains, "You will find rest for your souls. For my yoke is easy and my burden is light." We must learn how to give God our problems, and difficulties. When we do, he replaces our feelings of anxiety with peacefulness. We know we can't change the situation, but he can.

One night before I left for a trip, the circuit breaker for my pool pump quit working. What in the world could I do? The electrician and pool businesses were closed. In the Florida heat, my pool would turn green without water circulation while I was away.

That evening, I prayed and asked God to be with me as I tried to resolve the situation. I handed my problem to the Lord and had faith that he would show me what to do. He had previously helped me through much worse situations. I did not lose sleep that night worrying.

In the morning, while at the airport, I left a message at the electrician's office. They notoriously did not respond for weeks as a rule, as they were so busy with new construction. After the call, I prayed, asked for God's favor, and boarded my flight. During my layover, to my surprise, the company's receptionist called me and said they would have an electrician at my house by one p.m. Wow, I had put my faith in God and another issue resolved easily.

When we worry, stress-response hormones are released. Therefore, as soon as we recognize our focus is on the negative, we should pray. We can actually change our thoughts by focusing on God and asking him to solve our problem. This type of praying will give us God's peace. We need to put the issue in his hands and meditate on a Bible verse. By using scripture, we retrain our minds to remove harmful thoughts.

If something worries me, I pray about it every time the thought enters my mind—like waiting for biopsy results. Instead of fearing a potential undesirable outcome, I think of God and pray. I train my mind to bring every destructive thought to God.

Second Corinthians 10:5 teaches us, "We demolish arguments and every pretension that sets itself up against the knowledge of God, and we take captive every thought to make it obedient to Christ" (NIV). I used the strategy from this verse to train my mind to bring every negative thought to Jesus and ask him to remove it and replace it with a truth from his Word. This tactic works. Next time you experience undesirable thoughts, tell God how you feel and ask him to help you replace your thoughts with positive ones. You can renew your mind (replace negative thoughts with positive ones) through the Word of God.

Philippians 4:6–7 says, "Don't worry about anything; instead, pray about everything. Tell God what you need and thank him for all he has done. Then you will experience God's peace, which exceeds anything we can understand. His peace will guard your hearts and minds as you live in Christ Jesus." From this verse, I created a stress relief formula.

Don't Worry + Pray + Thank God + Abide in Christ = God's Peace

When you worry, pray and thank God in advance for his answers. Cast that worry from your mind into God's capable arms. Thank him for what you have. What does it mean to abide in Christ? You abide in Jesus when you do the following:

- Follow the Holy Spirit's direction as you sense it.
- Talk to Jesus throughout the day.
- Ask him to support you in your daily challenges.
- Listen to the Spirit's quiet guidance.

I pray you will use God's stress relief formula to enhance the peace you feel in your heart. Tapping into his power will help you make better choices to manage your anxiety and persevere when tempted to get stress relief from the wrong sources or to let worry create further ongoing anxiety.

When an anxious thought pops up—pray. Take your problems to the Lord and ask him to help you. Have faith that he will. Every time you dread an issue, speak this Bible verse out loud, "You will keep in perfect peace all those whose thoughts are fixed on you!" (Isaiah 26:3). When you memorize scripture, you can call upon God's supernatural power to help you.

MEMORIZE SCRIPTURE

Find a Bible verse you can relate to, write it down, and memorize it. God's Word is part of your spiritual arsenal that you can unsheathe and use as an offensive weapon to remove negative thoughts plaguing your mind.

Memorizing scripture reduces stress and temptation (like the desire to eat sugary, unhealthy food). Here are some helpful hints to memorize Bible verses:

1. Write the Bible verse down on an index card or some other form of paper. Write the scripture reference (that is, Isaiah 26:3) at the top and bottom of the card and the verse in between. When writing the verse, break it up into short segments that are easier to memorize.
2. Learn one line of the verse at a time but always start with the reference name and number because it is harder to remember that than the actual verse. Continue to practice until you have the full verse memorized.
3. Put the Bible verse in a common place like on your refrigerator door, bathroom mirror, or car dashboard. After you've learned it, review it a couple times a month to keep it vivid in your mind.

Then you can call upon God's powerful words at any time. God spoke the entire world into existence. His words are authoritative. Speak the verse out loud with confidence. In the spiritual realm, the spoken Word of God unsheathes the sword of the Spirit and has power over unseen forces influencing the mind and body. Use God's powerful weapon.

RELATIONAL BOUNDARIES

Another major stressor in life is our relationships. And we can often be blind to how much relational stress is depleting our physical and emotional health. Often only intentional self-examination can assess the harmony and disharmony in our lives.

Be willing to take a hard look at how you interact with people in your life. Which relationships cause you stress? For me, it was my aunt. Make a list of the people who bring you peace and those who cause you anxiety. Do some friends or family members deplete you versus build you up? If yes, it is time to set boundaries with those relationships. What can you do to minimize these stressful situations?

Earlier in my life, when my mother upset me, I would talk with my two sisters about her behind her back. The book *Boundaries* by Drs. Henry Cloud and John Townsend helped me develop personal boundaries by teaching me to go directly to the person I had an issue with.[10] The Bible directs us to do that too: "If another believer sins against you, go privately and point out the offense. If the other person listens and confesses it, you have won that person back" (Matthew 18:15).

I decided to try this approach. I explained to my mother what she did to upset me. What happened next surprised me. My mother apologized. Instead of creating a triangle of gossip with my sisters, I resolved the situation with my mother directly. It worked.

Boundaries are like fences. You want to keep beneficial people inside your fence and harmful ones outside. We have a responsibility to set limits for what we will allow, and we have the power to minimize the negative behavior others put on us. We have to figure out how. Brainstorm how to decrease the time you spend with those who harm you.

Heated interactions with others may cause the body to release cortisol and epinephrine. We want to minimize these types of interactions because, when they become chronic, they are harmful.[11] Establishing boundaries with others will help us do that.

We have accountability for our own conduct too. We should act honorably and treat others with respect, as we would want them to treat us. However, God does not want his children to be harmed by others, so establish your limits around negative influencers and stick with those boundaries.

Sometimes, however, we cause more stress through our own grudges and bitterness. If we harbor anger and resentment against others, the weight from it can shorten our lives. The opposite is true when we feel God's peace. This is the peace Jesus told us we couldn't get from this world. Thoughts and emotions can affect our anxiety level and overall health. Seek positive thinking and emotions. If needed, get counseling to help work through issues and set boundaries.

NAME, CLAIM, AND TAME IT

None of us gets out of this life without experiencing trauma. If a stressful situation triggers a past traumatic event, your body responds as if you were in that dreadful situation again.[12] Stress hormones are released, and your heart rate increases. Fear ensues, and you react negatively. This happens to all of us. But we can do something about it.

First, learn to realize when this happens and what triggers your return to a traumatic event. When I heard a car drive up that sounded similar to my ex-husband's vehicle, my heart pounded. I needed to understand what was happening. My mind would reel back in time to abusive situations. Instead, I needed to recognize that I was being triggered.

Once a person understands a trigger, they can name it, claim it, and tame it. Start by reminding yourself that you are not living in the past. The present moment is different; it is now, and you can tame the emotions that arise from a remembrance from the past. Objectify the feeling—name it—and put it in a mental arena where you can deal with it—tame it.

The next time you feel triggered, name what triggered you. Claim that the past is not a part of the current situation. Tame your response by speaking a Bible verse you memorized. Name, claim, and tame the trigger, and your response to it will improve.

This is another part of training the mind and bringing every negative thought captive to Christ (2 Corinthians 10:5). When you understand that you have been triggered, you can pray and ask God to take away the emotions from a perceived stress.

Once triggered, we may unintentionally lash out at loved ones. We do not want to harm others because we are reliving how someone, or something, harmed us in the past. Our emotions and thought life are a huge part of our inner being. We should seek therapy for past trauma. Counseling will improve our overall well-being and hopefully decrease the harmful reactions we may have toward others.

CHRISTIAN YOGA

Yoga reduces stress and exercises the body. I have been doing yoga since my twenties. For two decades, I've taught Scripture Yoga where I recite Bible verses while performing yoga poses. I've even published the books *Scripture Yoga* and *Yoga for Beginners.*

If you are concerned about yoga, please understand that people have been doing yoga since long before Hinduism (1500 BC[13]) and Buddhism (600 BC[14]) began their association with it. Stone seals that date back to 3000 BC were found with figures depicting yoga postures.[15] God knows who you worship. When we focus on God's truths as we seek physical relief from stress in yoga, we can sense his peace.

Yoga has many mental and physical benefits.[16] When you get into a yoga posture, you focus on your breathing and the sensations in your body. The breath slows down and becomes deeper, so you focus on the moment, which decreases stress. As muscles stretch, tension releases, and the mind becomes quiet, which allows worries to drift away. Performing yoga brings forth a peaceful state of mind and well-being.

Yoga helps you watch and regulate emotions.[17] During a yoga session, you learn to observe what you are thinking, and this helps prevent self-sabotaging thoughts. It's almost like being in cognitive behavioral therapy, but it doesn't cost much, except your time. Yoga decreases anxiety and depression, so you feel happier.[18]

In yoga, we practice mind-body hygiene as we look at our thoughts and evaluate how we communicate with others. This observation brings objectivity and can help with social interactions. Through observations, we can identify negative self-talk and replace it with positive thoughts. Yoga helps us to be less reactive and more self-reflective.[19] It is like attending a self-improvement class.

Yoga is therapeutic. In fact, trauma victims are now being treated with yoga therapy.[20] I rarely experience negative self-talk. I believe my thought life improved through yoga and training my mind to bring every thought captive to Christ.

What a blessing this physical, mental, and emotional practice has been to my life. When I added Bible verses to meditate upon during the sessions, this improved my spiritual life and helped me draw closer to God. Memorizing scripture helped place those Bible verses into my heart so I could draw upon them when needed. These Bible verses have helped me minister to others too.

A yoga session concludes with a time of meditation. Calming the mind with meditation through yoga is essential for stress management.[21] Many studies have found that mediation enhances concentration and memory.[22] We all need more of that. This meditative time also provides an opportunity for your mind to stop spinning so you can focus on the Lord. During this quiet time, it is easier to hear God's small, quiet voice.

I love the core strength obtained through yoga.[23] Muscle strength helps prevent injuries, especially as we age. Yoga is not competitive, so you do the class according to your abilities. Yoga is very accessible through classes at a gym, DVDs, and online streaming. Check out my Christian yoga DVDs at ChristianYoga.com. Your physical state need not deter you, as you can find many types of yoga classes and workshops in person or online, such as chair yoga, yoga for Parkinson's, yoga for cancer survivors, and so on. You can practice yoga your entire life, even into your centennial years.

Through yoga your emotional equilibrium stabilizes,[24] which improves self-control and helps control food cravings. Instead of grabbing some junk food, pull out your mat and do some yoga postures while reciting Bible verses. We each have the power to improve our health and life.

ADDITIONAL STRESS REDUCERS

Stress eating is common with many people. When we feel the pressure rise, we grab the chips and munch. Instead, we should turn to the Lord for his provision and cast our anxiety on him.

Stay away from social media as it can be such a downer and produce anxiety when we compare our lives with what we see on the screen. Social isolation, which occurs more as we age, can cause boredom and mindless eating. We eat without being hungry. When a person is bored, she may look in the refrigerator or pantry but can't find anything appealing. If this happens, drink two glasses of water, as you may be thirsty and don't realize it. Many seniors do not drink an adequate amount of water[25] (see chapter 2 for recommended water requirements).

When you recognize you are about to emotionally eat, do the following:

- Perform Christian yoga.
- Pray and express your emotions to God.
- Ask God to transform your mind.
- Recite a Bible verse out loud (put one on the refrigerator).
- Go on a walk.
- Call a friend.
- Journal.

You can also appease your emotional appetite by eating God's healthy foods. Make sure you have these nutritious foods on hand. Here are a few delicious examples:

- Eat raw nuts.
- Keep boiled eggs on hand.
- Try fresh fruit. Fruits are God's dessert.
- Add almond butter to each slice of a green apple. This treat tastes sweet, but it is high in protein.
- Create chocolate-covered nut clusters by melting 70 percent dark chocolate in a pan on the stove. Add nuts until well coated with the chocolate. Place mounds of nut clusters on wax paper.
- Eat dips like hummus or guacamole with a platter of fresh vegetables, such as cucumbers, celery, and carrots.

These techniques will help you break the cycle of emotional eating. Each time you recognize you're eating because of your emotions, use these tips to disengage the connection between food and feelings.

Many people have such high-paced lives that their bodies get stuck in the sympathetic mode (fight-or-flight), so it is difficult for them to relax (parasympathetic mode—rest/digest). One relaxation technique is the use of a sauna. Infrared saunas dilate the blood vessels and relax muscles through warmth, which puts you into the parasympathetic mode. When you step out of the sauna, you feel relaxed and content. Using the sauna regularly resets the body's balance between the two types of nervous systems to alleviate chronic tension.[26] If you don't have access to a sauna, do things that would cause you to sweat like working in the yard. Learn what other techniques help you relax your body and mind.

Some other positive coping strategies for dealing with stress are listed below:

- Exercise by doing an activity you enjoy.
- Sleep at least eight hours each night.
- Spend time with God every day, pray, and meditate with him.
- Determine three things you are grateful for before getting out of bed.
- Breathe deeply when you experience a challenging situation.
- Sing praise and worship songs when you shower.
- Tell yourself two or three positive traits about you.
- Hug yourself by grabbing your upper arms with your hands.
- Pet your animal.
- Hug your partner, grandchildren, or other kids in your life.

In life, we need to achieve balance. And managing stress is a big part of that, since we all experience it. We need to recognize when our body goes into the fight-or-flight response from perceived or noncritical reasons and stop that response by calming down. We can't incorporate all of these suggestions, but we can try to manage our stress and have a peaceful heart and mind through using some of the strategies in this chapter.

PERSONAL AND PRACTICAL APPLICATION

1. Were you surprised to find that stress does not cause ulcers but rather the gut bacterium H. pylori? Have you asked your doctor to test you for this harmful bacterium to avoid negative health issues caused by an imbalanced gut?
2. What stress symptoms do you suffer from? List them here.
3. What causes you stress? List your stressors here.

4. Have you found God's peace in your life? Do you cast your burdens and anxiety on him? What burden do you need to cast to the Lord right now?
5. Do you tend to be a worrier? If yes, what tactics will you use to reduce your anxiety?
6. What Bible verse would you like to memorize? Write it on a card so you can learn it.
7. What type of boundaries do you need to set and with whom?
8. Have you ever felt triggered because of a past situation? What was it? How can you learn to recognize those triggers in the future?
9. What techniques do you plan to use to reduce your stress?
10. Do you engage in relaxation techniques such as Christian yoga or meditation? What can you try to help you relax?
11. Do you tend to emotionally eat? What can you do reduce this behavior?

CHAPTER 8
MAINTAIN A POSITIVE EMOTIONAL LIFE

It's a wonderful thing to be optimistic. It keeps you healthy and it keeps you resilient.
—Daniel Kahneman

You can view life as either half full or half empty. While the circumstances might be the same either way, your attitude makes the distinction. And the difference between positive and negative can create a world of difference in the years you have left on this earth.

I wake up each morning with a positive attitude. For twenty-four years, I was married to a man who was the opposite. He constantly focused on the negative side of situations and how they could turn out worse.

As a mother of two young children, I learned to laugh at terrible situations in my life. Otherwise, I would've gone crazy or cried. One morning after getting my three-year-old and one-year-old dressed to go to the church nursery so I could attend a Bible study, a mess occurred. My baby was on my hip as I held my older daughter's hand. As we stepped into the garage, I felt something wet on my hip. I looked down to find my youngest had a bowel blowout all over my shirt and pants. What a smelly mess.

At that moment, I could either cry, laugh, or become angry. Ever since that experience, I have chosen to laugh in situations where I might normally scream. Life is full of messes. You probably encounter one every day. How we react to these messes will either hurt or help us deal with life's difficulties.

When you look at your mess from a humorous viewpoint, it brings a smile to your face. When you laugh at your own situations, your stress fades. Laughter makes it easier to cope with tough situations. It actually reduces the physical symptoms of stress and lessens depression and anxiety. Amusement makes you feel happier. Laughter is a healthy reaction we should elicit more often.

Next time you find a blowout dripping down your hip or some other calamity—laugh. Even if it feels forced at first, practice laughing. Really get into it and laugh harder and longer than you normally would. Laughing releases dopamine in your brain, which is a feel-good neurohormone that delivers a relaxed feeling.[1]

Do things to promote amusement in your life, such as watching a comedy. If you receive a funny card or run across a humorous cartoon, keep these items in a special place in your home. Read them when you need to lift your spirit.

I enjoy watching *America's Funniest Home Videos.* The mishaps that occur are hilarious. Internet or social media videos of animals can be cute and comical as well. Include humor in your life, and you will be a happier person.

ATTITUDE

Aging happens to all of us; it is a natural process we should embrace, even if we seek to age gracefully. Greet each new year with thankfulness because the Bible considers a long life to be a blessing. Don't look back on the past only to relive the good old days. Truly, they are not as good as we remember them since we have selective memories. Instead, we should embrace where we are now and look forward to the next decade of our lives and all the joy we will discover. Psalm 100:4 tells us, "Give thanks to him and praise his name."

As we age and experience limitations, we may feel frustrated and angry. Those negative emotions won't change anything. In fact, they will make us harder to live with and be around. Life still offers much to be grateful for in our later years.

While aging may bring about more limitations, don't focus on what was lost. We may not be able to do what we used to, but we can focus on what we can do, and even try something new. Learn to emphasize the positive, not the negative. We can switch an undesirable mindset to an optimistic one when we have a grateful heart. Consider journaling three things you are grateful for every day.

Use a gratitude journal or simply take time each day to thank God for what you have. I like to name items of gratitude at the end of each day while watching the sunset. Each evening, God gives us the most spectacular light show. I sit on my back porch and watch the day turn to evening and finally into night. During that time, I list ten things I am grateful for. My heart fills to the brim with joy because when we express gratitude, our bodies release beneficial endorphins.[2] With gratefulness, in addition to your own relaxed sense of peace, your witness to those around you as a faithful, contented person can have a significant impact.

Besides a grateful heart, we need to make sure we're not complaining about others or about the circumstances of life. The only constant in this earthly life is change. Throughout our lives we have experienced much change. We need to be careful not to get so set in our ways that we resist change. Culture and society shift—it always has. Stop complaining about change and see what you can learn from it and from younger generations.

Think of the hippies in the 1960s and what the older generation thought of them. Maybe you were one of those hippies. We should not be so critical and judgmental of younger people. Our elders probably had negative thoughts about us when we were young. Be careful not to become bitter and inflexible. Look for opportunities where you can encourage others. Look for the good instead of focusing on cultural changes.

As we age, we have spent a lifetime experiencing struggles with career, marriage, and parenting. We know the challenges of daily living in this sinful world. We should look for opportunities to teach and share with younger people. We shouldn't only associate with older people. Other believers who are struggling to follow Jesus need people to look up to who have been there before. We all need to know what faithfulness looks like at an older age. You could be the example others need.

Strive to be a person worth respecting and listening to. The Bible teaches us that the elderly are a valuable part of society. "Wisdom belongs to the aged, and understanding to the old" (Job 12:12). We have a lot to offer through our experience and wisdom. We need to positively influence the younger generation, not complain about them as others did about us when we were young.

Consider how you can serve God in the situation you find yourself in today. Ultimately, we should seek ways to glorify God and honor him through our lives. Age should not be an excuse. If you have drifted away from your church, look for ways to become involved. Community is vital throughout our entire life, especially spiritual community. We will further discuss the benefits of community in chapter 10.

PROMOTE A POSITIVE MENTAL OUTLOOK

The best way to keep positive is through a dedicated, daily devotional time with the Lord. Take a few minutes to spend with him. You could read a devotion, Bible passage, or a scripture verse. After reading, meditate by focusing on your breath. Notice your chest rise with each deep inhalation. Allow divine thoughts to enter your mind. Mentally speak out a Bible verse you just read, over and over as you breathe. You can be so busy you are not still long enough to hear God speak. But meditating with the Lord like this allows God to penetrate your busy mind. Listen for God's quiet voice.

In addition to connecting with God and gratitude, other practices can increase your positive emotions. Spend time with emotionally fulfilling friends or family too. Share what is going on in your life and listen to them as well. Sharing our ups and downs, encouraging each other, and laughing with others brings the heart joy. These beneficial emotions fill us with a sense of well-being. That's what happens when you're with people who fill your emotional tank. Avoid those who deplete you.

Make sure you're getting enough sleep and not eating too much junk food. What you eat affects your mental outlook. It's easy to stay up late, race from one activity to another, and fill up with fast food, never realizing the toll it's taking on your emotions. You are more likely to make better choices and stay optimistic when your body is fed and rested properly.

Schedule time to do things you love. Take a walk in the park, listen to your favorite music, or go to the movies. Whatever brings you happiness or creates a positive attitude.

I thoroughly enjoy spending time in nature. It resets my brain. Research has proven that "forest bathing" (spending time in nature while paying attention to the five senses) improves a person's overall well-being.[3] While you walk in the woods, listen to the bird's chirp, smell the flowers or freshly mowed grass, and feel the wind against your skin. Spending time in nature restores the body through effortless attention to what God has placed around us. God gave us nature to help regulate our emotions by calming our soul. He made the forest for us to enjoy, and it restores us physically and psychologically, which is absolutely amazing!

Hundreds of research studies have proven the benefits of forest bathing and found it improves the following:[4]

- well-being
- emotions
- depression
- mood disorders
- overall health
- immune system
- high blood pressure
- prosocial helping behaviors
- prefrontal cortex of the brain
- mental relaxation and decreased stress and anxiety
- function of the cardiovascular and respiratory systems

Forest bathing reduces mental health symptoms and, in particular, anxiety. So, when you experience tension, take a break by going outside. You could sit on your porch or take a short walk around your home. While you do, feel the breeze or the heat of the sun and listen to the birds sing. I believe time in nature restores and reverses the harmful mental and physical effects of technology that constantly bombard our senses.

Two of the most calming colors to the mind and spirit are green and blue.[5] Maybe that is why God made the skies blue and the foliage green. These soothing colors that we find outside harmonize the soul. Try to spend at least fifteen minutes a day in nature.

These techniques will increase your positive emotions. Find ways to overcome negativity, cope with stress, and create helpful emotions in your life.

MINDSET MANAGEMENT

Our thought life is more important than we might imagine. You can change the character of your life through your thoughts and beliefs. Some views are self-limiting. Recognize and change them.

Science now understands that our genes turn on or off through environmental effects. Part of that includes our thoughts, attitude, and mindset. Positive thoughts have a profound impact on our genes. Negative thoughts have an equally powerful effect. Thoughts influence the expression of genes.[6]

To ensure optimism, you can change your thoughts, attitude, and mindset, even if you've always thought, *That's just the way I am*. Managing your mind is part of living a healthy lifestyle with less stress, anxiety, and more happiness. You want to increase your positive emotions, but pessimistic thoughts may continue to harass you. Undesirable thoughts feed destructive emotions. What can you do to prevent the downward spiral of negativity?

You have more power than you think. Remember how we looked at 2 Corinthians 10:5 in chapter 7 when we talked about worry. This verse reminds us to "take captive every thought to make it obedient to Christ" (NIV). While we know this means to replace negative thinking when we begin to worry, what Paul said goes even further. You can actually monitor what's going on in your mind. But how do you take unwanted thoughts captive? These steps will help:

1. Notice your thoughts. Most of them are on autopilot.
2. Determine if the thought is beneficial or harmful.

3. Check the negative thought against reality. Is it true or false? If it is false, recognize it. Journal the belief and how it is not true.
4. If the thought is harmful, direct it in a more positive direction through reframing your thought. Reframing allows you to take a bad thought and make it positive. For example, you notice a family member did not do a chore you asked them to perform. Instead of feeling frustrated, you could reframe your original thought into something like, *I'm so thankful they are in my life.* The new, reframed thought gives a sense of gratitude and love, which generates healthier emotions. The circumstances didn't change, but the way you thought about them did.
5. Ask God to take the negative thought away from you.
6. Recite a Bible verse that counters the destructive thought. Whenever the pestering belief returns, speak that verse out loud, and stab the unwanted spiritual influence with the sword of the Spirit.

These techniques reduce stress and anxiety and promote positive feelings. We will experience more encouraging emotions as we manage our minds. When we feel good, we act in beneficial ways. Use these steps to overcome negativity. Practice them until they become second nature. You will enjoy a healthier life when you do.

PURPOSE AND SERVICE

Finding purpose in our senior years is essential to our well-being. When we don't have a sense of purpose, we lose motivation for other aspects of life. When we lose a source of meaning in our lives, we are at risk for mental health issues such as depression. A sedentary life also leads to a decline in physical abilities and stamina.

During transitional times of life, we may experience empty-nest syndrome as the kids leave or a loss of identity as we retire from a job. Empty-nest syndrome is the sadness or emotional distress we feel when our children grow up and leave home. With these changes, we experience mixed emotions. These are some thoughts I experienced: *Finally, after twenty-five years, I've got my life back. I don't have to cook and clean for my kids anymore. But what am I going to do now? Am I still valuable? Are my kids okay?*

We may also experience grief, depression, and loss of purpose. We should allow ourselves to experience those emotions. If we don't know what it feels like to be sad, how can we experience true happiness? God gave us emotions and tears. Crying is God's way of removing our sadness. When you feel like crying, cry. When I do, I like to sob into my pillow. I really let it out. Afterward, I feel lighter—like I'm carrying less emotional baggage.

Besides feeling our emotions, we should try to understand them. Yes, it made sense for me to feel sad when each of my children left home. I even wore black for several weeks to express outwardly how I felt inwardly. But after a period of time, we need to find a new purpose and let the sun shine on our emotions. It is not emotionally healthy to partake in a pity party for an extended length of time. If we don't recover within a few months, we should seek counseling.

When we reach a point in life where our lives and schedules slow down, we need some time to let our bodies recover from the decades of a fast-paced lifestyle. Then we need to find a new purpose. How can we serve others? What do we find fulfilling?

What divine purpose does the Lord have for you at this time in your life? Pray and ask God to reveal this to you. Meditate with the Lord to give him an opportunity to speak to you through your mind and his Holy Spirit.

The Bible does not designate a retirement period. In fact, the Bible indicates that the older, wiser generation should mentor the younger. That's our responsibility. How can we help those younger than us with the wisdom we've gained in our lives?

In today's world, in this country, retirement is part of the culture, but it was not prior to a century ago. Retirement with a Social Security pension was not introduced in the United States until 1935 by President Franklin D. Roosevelt.

We have more time in our retirement years than we have had in decades. We shouldn't sit around all day watching television. Yes, some downtime is restorative to the soul, but so is reading a book, working out at the gym, attending a Bible study, or socializing with a small group. Maybe you want to focus on your yard, flower beds, or vegetable garden. Gardening is great exercise, and it calms the soul.

Seniors are valuable to society. We are full of wisdom from the tough lives we've lived. Our experiences can help others. If we knew what we know now when we were teens, we would have lived a better life. We can use our value to serve others.

You may have not gotten to choose the most satisfying job previously, but you can now. Take a spiritual gifts test and find your strengths if you don't know them already. When you figure out what you excel in and have confidence in those strengths, you will shine. Try different forms of service in the church or community. The options are endless. Hospitals love volunteers, but so do nonprofit organizations.

I tried working in the church nursery, but it gave me a headache. Through singing in the church choir, I realized I couldn't carry a tune. However, I enjoyed teaching women's Bible studies. That was not surprising once I found out my spiritual gift was teaching. When you apply your God-given gifts, the task becomes much easier.

If you love animals, check out opportunities at animal shelters, or you could foster an animal until it has a permanent home. You could do the same for children and become a foster parent. Food pantries and homeless shelters always need help. You could bring residents at a senior living facility joy by volunteering your time or talents.

You could also take a mission trip with your church or a nonprofit. Going to another region to assist others helps us appreciate the small things in life and shifts our focus from ourselves. I went on five mission trips to Ecuador when my daughters were teenagers. One year I led a group of teens and adults. All participants grew in community and wisdom as we worked to raise money and learned about a new culture.

Serving the impoverished broadens our life perspective. Many teens were perplexed over how those poverty-stricken Ecuadorian children were so happy with so little, while they had so much. After returning from the trip, simple things became more satisfying.

If you need to continue to work, explore new employment options. I started a new career in my midfifties as an author. Previously, I was a nurse and health care administrator. But I felt a calling on my life

Maintain a Positive Emotional Life

to write about healthy living topics with a Christian slant. Has God placed a book in your heart to write?

Employment opportunities are endless. Explore. See what you find that appeals to you. AARP and other senior living organizations offer many opportunities to discover both new hobbies and new areas of employment. Match your strength and passion with your new purpose. Maybe you've always loved teens and have a desire to inspire them. Volunteer at your church's youth group or become a scout leader. Many choices are available for you to discover.

The intrinsic feeling from serving others through employment or volunteering is phenomenal. Positive endorphins are released, and you feel satisfied. You walk away knowing you did your part to make this a better world.

The options for your life's purpose in this new phase of life are numerous. Switch the "poor me" attitude of loss for the upbeat attitude of what a child experiences when they walk into a candy store and get to choose one item. What will they choose? That is you. Have fun deciding. Maybe you can taste a few pieces of candy before selecting.

COUNSELING

When we find purpose, we feel more valuable; yet that's only part of the puzzle of how we see ourselves. Beliefs influence decisions. What do you believe about yourself? Negative feelings about self-image affect self-worth. Do you focus on the lies of the Enemy, or does the Holy Spirit lead you to trust that you do not have a spirit of fear and timidity but a spirit of power, love, and a sound mind (2 Timothy 1:7)? What you choose to put into your mind is key to creating a positive and healthy belief system. You'll only be able to continue to walk in your new purpose if you believe you are worthy of it and still have much to contribute.

As your physical, mental, and emotional habits improve, your self-respect should too. There is a correlation between how you think of yourself and how you take care of your body and spirit. If you're not taking care of yourself, figure out why. What is the emotional reason? Does it have to do with your identity? Do you experience self-hatred? If so, see a therapist.

If you have not been practicing health habits for a long time, a counselor can help you determine the root reason why. Maybe you have unresolved trauma, which resulted in negative self-talk and loathing. Get some emotional support to understand the underlying reason you're not taking care of yourself. When you respect and believe in yourself, your health habits improve.

Most of us should receive counseling at some point in our lives. As Jesus said, here on earth you will have many trials and sorrows, and we do. Whether it is from trauma, abuse, or other ordeals, it's therapeutic to speak with a counselor. If you prefer, seek out a Christian counselor who understands your spiritual identity in the Lord. We should never feel weird or shameful in talking to a trained professional. Sharing our feelings helps us heal. Proverbs 17:22 states, "A cheerful heart is good medicine, but a broken spirit saps a person's strength."

If you sustained some sort of trauma, and most of us have, desensitization therapies are available. After therapy, you won't continue to relive the trauma or feel those feelings when you get triggered by a current-day event.

We don't get through this life unscathed. Any given day can bring a form of abuse and trauma—emotional, physical, financial, neglect, abandonment, sexual, and so on. So what do we do with the unwanted emotional baggage? We work to heal our invisible wounds.

After my divorce from my abusive husband of twenty-four years, I knew I'd been harmed emotionally. With low self-esteem and a broken heart, I sought treatment. First, I went through four months of a Breaking Free course along with bimonthly group therapy. This course helped me break the cyclical bond of abuse.

Next, I received group therapy from Leslie Vernick, the Christian author of *The Emotionally Destructive Marriage*. I learned abuse patterns to make sure I never fell into this form of mistreatment again. Slowly, my mindset improved from negative to positive.

After that, I took an online course for those who've been emotionally abused. This was the best and least expensive treatment. The course suggested that each participant write their abuser(s) a note or pretend to speak to them. Then you tell them how they hurt you. This assignment was to be completed for each abuser—as there is usually more than one.

I followed the instructions provided in the course. I sat down and pretended my abuser was sitting across from me. I explained what he or she did and how it made me feel and how it would affect me for the rest of my life. With each abuser, I cried and wailed until there were no tears left. The next step was to forgive each individual who harmed me. With God's help, I did. The relief and feeling of lightness in my heart after I did was unbelievable. It was like darkness left and light permeated my entire being. And that light brought me profound joy.

I can't express how therapeutic this process was for me. Do you need to forgive someone? Trauma leaves a devastating mark on a person's life, and all of us have been traumatized. Each of us needs to seek therapy for the traumas we've sustained in our life.

But I wasn't done yet. I wanted to make sure I received a significant amount of mental health treatment to make sure that any future partner would not receive the brunt of my issues. I wanted to heal, so I saw a Christian counselor for the next year and a half. At the end of that time, the counselor said, "Susan, you don't feel anger, hatred, or animosity toward your ex-husband. I don't think we need to continue your counseling anymore. You have a healed heart." Wow, that was amazing to hear.

My carefree heart was joyful. I regained my self-confidence and sought a new career as a Christian author. I felt this was my God-given mission, which my ex-husband did not want me to pursue. I was healed. Now I am happier than I have been in years. I am following God's plan for my life. His path for me is better than anything I could have imagined.

INTERPERSONAL RELATIONSHIPS

Relationships with others can be filled with strife. The arena of interpersonal relationships is one of the most challenging spiritual battlegrounds we face. Paul explains this in Ephesians 4:26–27: "And 'don't sin by letting anger control you.' Don't let the sun go down while you are still angry, for anger gives a foothold to the devil." When we remain angry at someone who has offended or sinned against us, we allow a door of opportunity for Satan to influence us.

Harmful thoughts swirl in our minds as we fume. That is why Paul recommends we don't let anger cause us to act sinfully in return, and we reconcile before the day is over. Paul suggests we forgive the person before we go to sleep. Have you ever lost sleep from angry thoughts churning in your mind? I have—many times. When we forgive, then Satan doesn't have access to our minds.

Satan's schemes involve anger, unforgiveness, and bitterness. He desires broken relationships with friends, family members, and communities like churches. Unforgiveness toward a person gives the devil an opportunity to influence you. For that reason, Paul explains in 2 Corinthians 2:10–11, "And when I forgive whatever needs to be forgiven, I do so with Christ's authority for your benefit, so that Satan will not outsmart us. For we are familiar with his evil schemes."

It is impossible to fully love God and commune with him while harboring hatred for another. Harboring hatred and bitterness harm your psychological well-being. Do you have someone in your life you need to forgive? I did. What a relief when I finally forgave. Unforgiveness harms the person who does not forgive. You might think it harms the person who wronged you, but it doesn't. Sometimes I have to ask God to help me forgive because I can't do it on my own. Ask him and he will help you forgive too.

What if you wronged someone in your life? What should you do? The Old Testament provides an example. In Genesis 27, we find the story of two brothers, Esau and Jacob. Jacob stole Esau's blessing when he disguised himself as his brother and asked their dying father to bless him instead of the oldest—Esau. Ultimately, Jacob fled Israel after his father died, so Esau would not murder him.

Decades later, Jacob returned to Israel and knew he must face his brother for his deceit. Jacob lived with that nagging sin in his heart for years. He was scared to face Esau, but when he did, Jacob bowed, offered bountiful gifts, and apologized. Jacob did all of this to make restitution for what he stole. Jacob's actions softened Esau's heart, and they reconciled. After all those years, Jacob finally felt peace in his heart for settling his wrongdoing with his brother.

Is there someone you need to forgive or reconcile with? Pray and ask God how you should proceed. We face more than just death at the end of our life. We will face the judgment seat of God. Be sure to forgive and make amends with others while you are still living.

Changing our negative mindset and undesirable habits to healthy habits begins in the mind. If we understand what caused our pessimistic mindset, we can rewire our brain to be optimistic. This goes for thoughts about self, food, and healthy habits. Positivity will keep you healthier as you age.

PERSONAL AND PRACTICAL APPLICATION

1. Do you have an optimistic or pessimistic attitude? If pessimistic, what techniques will you try to change it?
2. Are you guilty of grumbling about the younger generation? What can you do to positively affect someone younger?
3. How do you practice gratitude? What can you do to enhance your gratefulness?
4. What do you like to do for fun? When was the last time you engaged in a fun activity?
5. Do you need to change your mindset? What strategy will you use to change it?
6. Does your life have purpose? If not, what can you do to regain that purpose?
7. Do you work or volunteer? If not, pray and ask God if and where you should.
8. Have you ever received counseling? If not, do you have past trauma or abuse that needs healing?
9. Do you need to forgive someone? If yes, how can you proceed?
10. Do you need to reconcile a wrong you did earlier in your life? How can you reconcile?

CHAPTER 9
GUARD YOUR MENTAL HEALTH

> *Wellness is the complete integration of body, mind, and spirit—the realization that everything we do, think, feel, and believe has an effect on our state of well-being.*
>
> —Greg Anderson

As we age, we face new and potentially life-changing challenges. Retiring from a career brings major concerns, such as: Will I have enough income? Will Medicare adequately cover my health expenses? And more health issues arise as we get older because our bodies naturally degenerate and ultimately pass away. No matter what, we all die. We can't stop this natural process, but by applying the techniques in this book, we can slow the aging process and look forward to our everlasting life with the Lord.

In chapter 8, we discussed attitude. Think about two people looking at the same scenario: one may see a cup half full, while the other sees it half empty. Our attitude toward retirement and an empty nest can be viewed as losing one's identity versus changing it. For many people, their self-worth is closely related to their career or parenthood. However, you can change your priorities.

Once you determine what fulfills you in this chapter of your life, it can give you a new purpose. Have you wanted to travel more or pursue a creative outlet? Maybe you can finally spend more time with family and friends or frequent a health club. We discussed many potential new purposes in the last chapter. In this one, there are many issues we need to address to prepare our mental health for the golden years.

MENTAL HEALTH STRESSORS

During this transitional time, there are numerous major life changes that may occur causing mental health issues to arise. Closing one chapter of our life through retirement is just one scenario. Some of the additional stressors include a chronic illness, moving, or losing a spouse. We can feel uncertainty and fear as we adjust. Some changes are expected—like moving—others are not.

Relationships

You might have more time to manage your relationships now. Relationships take work, so focus on the most important ones. Spending time with family and friends cultivates closeness.

Identify and disengage from toxic relationships. If this is a family member, it is more difficult to do. But you can figure out ways to navigate this avenue strategically.

Establishing healthy boundaries and negotiating reasonable expectations with loved ones is always beneficial. For example, does your son have a long list of projects he wants you to complete? Or is your daughter waiting for you to retire so you can be her children's full-time babysitter? If that's what you want—great! Just realize that this kind of commitment will limit your ability to fulfill yourself in other ways. More significantly, resulting resentment may harm your relationship with family members. Learn to say no when needed. It is challenging to accept our adult children's decisions and how they choose to raise their children, especially when we do not approve. Instead of creating conflict, we can pray for them and our grandchildren.

Be open to new friendships, no matter what your age. When you are involved in activities and attend events, opportunities arise where you meet others. Occasionally, you feel a kindred friendship with someone new. Take the next step and invite them to join you for lunch. Cultivating new friendships promotes a positive mental outlook.

My ninety-year-old mother-in-law walks two miles daily in her neighborhood and has done so for the past seventeen years. She and her husband downsized and moved to this new home and neighborhood in their seventies. He died seven years ago.

Recently she shared how the relationships she's created through her walks helped her not be isolated after her husband's death. She spoke with many neighbors as the occasion arose during her walks. She's watched neighborhood kids grow up and has felt a connection with others. Human interaction is vital for our mental well-being. Make sure you stay engaged with others. Don't climb into a shell of isolation.

Loss

As we age, we may lose our spouse through divorce or death, which creates an extremely challenging time of our life—heart wrenching, in fact. It can wreak havoc on your mental health. But we can endure, especially if we lean on God. During the year of my divorce, I recited Matthew 6:34, "So don't ever worry about tomorrow. . . . Each day has enough trouble of its own" (GW). Every time I thought about the future, I recited that verse, and it helped me focus on what I had to deal with that day. Ask God for a specific Bible verse to help you get through a tough time.

Besides the heartfelt loss, there is so much responsibility to deal with after a loved one dies. The list below shows the huge amount of work that is thrust upon the surviving spouse.

- funeral arrangements
- will, trust, estate arrangements
- asset distribution to heirs
- probate
- notification of family, friends, employer, banks, credit cards, financial institutions, insurance companies, and so on
- survivor Social Security benefits
- cancellation of services like cell phones, streaming devices, and so on
- debt payment or forgiveness arrangements
- property and income taxes
- distribution and removal of personal belongings
- car title and tag changes

The list goes on and on and can be overwhelming. I remember how hard it was for my aunt to handle all the responsibilities thrust upon her after my uncle died, especially since she had never dealt with the financial obligations of the household. Her daughter helped her through that tumultuous ordeal.

All of us leave behind a life that must be closed. If your spouse dies, all those legal and personal details are left for you to handle. It's an enormous responsibility to deal with while you are grieving. Therefore, advanced planning is essential.

Get your estate documents developed or updated. Visit an attorney and have them create your will or trust. Make a list of your passwords and keep them with your will so your family can easily cancel subscriptions and such. Keep your medication list and copies of insurance cards updated and in a visible place easily found. Make sure your family knows where you store essential documents. When my adult children come home to visit, I make sure they know where my trust, passwords, and essential documents are in my home.

If your loved one suffers from dementia or some other disabling disease and you do not want resuscitation by emergency medical professionals, place the Do Not Resuscitate order (DNR) on the refrigerator. During an emergency, after you've called an ambulance is not the time to locate this documentation.

Immediately after a loved one dies is not a good time to make major life-changing decisions. I remember my parents discussing these types of decisions when my father was diagnosed with cancer. He told my mom not to make any huge changes, like moving, until one year after he had passed. That way her mental outlook on life would hopefully be more balanced.

When a loved one dies, your mental world is placed into a raging sea. End-of-life planning will make the sea calmer for the person left behind. Strengthen your ability to cope with life by preplanning.

Funeral Planning

Plan your funeral before you die. Make arrangements at a funeral home or mortuary. Will you be cremated, or do you need to choose your casket? Purchase your burial plot or urn. Pick out the Bible passages, songs, pallbearers, a eulogy speaker, and so on. Write the newspaper notification and eulogy. Keep this documentation in the same place as your will.

My brother shared with me his desired arrangements. He wants us to rent a party boat and sprinkle his ashes in the Gulf of Mexico. What a fun way to remember him and celebrate his life. My sister-in-law only wants a quiet family service. Each of us is different. Make your desires known before you pass away.

If you do not have any family members, who will you entrust? Who will you list on your will? Determining these issues is helpful for those left behind.

Grief Counseling

In addition to preplanning, grief counseling and support groups help a widow or widower after their spouse dies. The surviving spouse experiences a mixture of emotions. Those emotions should not be ignored but felt and managed. Family and friends can be a wonderful support, but possibly more is needed.

Working through the stages of grief (denial, anger, bargaining, depression, and acceptance) is vital to a person's mental well-being. Some who mourn may move into serious depression, which needs treatment. Therapy with a counselor can help one accept the death of a loved one, move through the stages of grief, and start a new life.

Support groups provide a means to share your feelings with others who are also grieving. Getting out of the house and interacting with others who can understand your feelings provides the needed emotional assistance. You can find support groups in your community through churches, funeral homes, hospitals, hospice, or your doctor.

Declutter

Rid your home of clutter. I've lived in my home for almost thirty years. A couple of years ago, for my birthday, my daughters gave me the book *The Life-Changing Magic of Tidying Up: The Japanese Art of Decluttering and Organizing.*[1] With this method, you look at each item in your home and decide if you receive pleasure from it as you choose to keep it or not.

I got the hint. I cleaned every closet in the house and removed vanloads of stuff. I donated it to a local charity for their garage sale. You could host your own yard sale if you wanted.

When I painted my house, I got rid of extra furniture I no longer needed. I gave an antique chair, given to me by my mother-in-law, to a niece, so it stayed in the family. My niece was thrilled and sent me a picture of it in her home.

My daughter helped me clean the garage—what a mess. Having someone else help you tackle an extensive project may give you the motivation needed to get the job done. Hiring someone to assist you is also an option. I've always asked the youth director at my church, "Which teenager needs to make money to attend a retreat or mission trip?" The director knows the kids and their families. Numerous young men and women have helped me garden, clean my garage, and keep up my yard through the years.

After my mother passed, I cleaned her closet. She had so many clothes. Did she need that many outfits? Check your closet. Are you keeping items you haven't worn for thirty years? It may be time to donate them. Remember, loved ones will be burdened with cleaning what you have left behind, so declutter.

Chronic Illness

Chronic diseases are conditions that last for over a year, and some for a lifetime. Most require ongoing medical attention and cause a person to limit their activities. Over 80 percent of seniors suffer from a chronic illness. Focusing on disease prevention, health promotion, and early detection are the best strategies.

Work with a trusted health care provider who can guide your education about the condition. Learning how to manage and improve the illness will help you develop coping skills to thrive in the face of your ailment.

The psychological effects of dealing with a chronic disease are tumultuous. You may question why you've been afflicted with it. Or you may feel shame that your lifestyle choices contributed to it. You may experience psychological issues as you deal with these feelings.

We can improve many chronic conditions by following the guidelines provided in this book. Lowering one's weight and blood sugar levels improves diabetes, high blood pressure, cardiovascular disease, and many other chronic conditions.[2] But if changing your lifestyle was easy to do, we would all do it. That is why I wrote *7 Steps to Get Off Sugar and Carbohydrates* from a Christian perspective to give the reader spiritual resources to make lasting lifestyle changes.

Many chronic conditions can be treated at one's home through home health care for nursing, physical therapy, and other services. We want to prolong one's residence in their own home.

Hospice treated my mother in her home during the last two years of her life. We no longer had to take her to the doctor; the hospice physician visited her. The biweekly aides helped care for her. This relieved my sister, who was the primary caregiver twenty-four hours a day. If you are a caregiver, it is vital to care for yourself and find community resources to help you bear the burden.

There are several resources to help individuals deal with chronic conditions.

- Program to Encourage Active, Rewarding Lives (PEARLS) at https://depts.washington.edu/hprc/programs-tools/pearls/
- Chronic Disease Self-Management Program (CDSMP) at https://chronicdisease.org
- The Multiple Chronic Conditions Resource Center offers free resources at https://multiplechronicconditions.org/patient-portal/

When a chronic disease strikes, you may need to think about your current home. Will it continue to serve you if you (or your spouse) develop a significant disability, such as the inability to climb stairs? Do you need to renovate or move? Adding grab bars to the shower and tub is an easy modification.

Many seniors downsize to a smaller home. They no longer need a big house, now that their children have left home. You may need to consider moving to an assisted living center.

Some people are very opposed to this option, while others are not. I've told my children that it is perfectly fine for me to move to one of those centers when the time comes. I am an extrovert and would enjoy meeting other residents. I think the games and activities of people my age would be entertaining.

Don't manage all of these changes on your own. Ask for help from loved ones and find community resources. You may need someone to drive you to an appointment or help with grocery shopping. My mother-in-law's sister could no longer drive due to macular degeneration. They asked me if I knew of anyone who could drive her to doctor's appointments and such. I did. A friend of mine was hired for the job, and this employment arrangement worked exceptionally well. Ask for assistance when needed.

Assistance

Communicate with your family and friends about your needs. Others don't know you need help unless you tell them. Do you need help cleaning the attic or picking up a prescription? Ask for support as needed. Don't allow yourself to become isolated. All of us need help sometimes.

Stubbornly refusing support can cause broken bones, unsafe homes, or poor mental and physical health from isolation. One fall could land you in a nursing home. Do you know of anyone that this has happened to?

It doesn't mean you are weak when you ask for assistance. It shows courage and responsibility. Asking can keep you healthier and more connected to others. Many people, like volunteers in your community, are pleased to support seniors. The hospice volunteers who watched my mother once a week, while my sister went grocery shopping, were lifesavers. These volunteers felt good about their contribution.

Identify who is best to call if needed. Many of us would call family first, but your adult child, with their own family, may live fifteen hundred miles away. So who can be relied upon when you need something? Figure this out. Research community and church resources and ask your physician.

Over time chronic disabilities are linked to loss of independence and social isolation, which affects one's mental health. Grief, loneliness, and major life changes can become deeper psychological issues. It is vital to understand how to manage mental health conditions, such as depression and anxiety, which may emerge during this transitional phase of life. Share how you feel with others and get the support you need.

Depression

Older adults are at an increased risk of depression during this time of life. Depression is a treatable medical condition, but it is not a normal part of aging.[3] Sometimes it's hard to tell if you have the blues or real depression.

When someone has other illnesses or limited function, they are more likely to experience depression, making this diagnosis more common among older adults.[4] When those feelings of sadness or anxiety last for weeks that turn into months—that's when you know something is wrong. When someone is depressed, they may experience the following:[5]

- pessimism
- worthlessness
- irritability
- hopelessness
- lower energy
- insomnia
- indecisiveness
- digestive issues
- overeating or loss of appetite
- difficulty concentrating
- loss of interest in activities that they previously enjoyed

Many may see their mood as a response to their life changes, but it may be depression. Therefore, they do not seek treatment. If you've suffered with many of the symptoms listed above for over a month, discuss this with your doctor. Medications and counseling help, as well as a healthy diet.

If you are reluctant to take medication, you could try a natural supplement that helps boost mood. Mayo Clinic cited the following supplements to help with depression:[6]

- Saint-John's-Wort
- S-adenosylmethionine (SAMe)
- omega-3 fatty acids
- 5-Hydroxytryptophan (5-HTP)
- dehydroepiandrosterone (DHEA)

You could try one of these supplements. If it does not relieve your symptoms, try another one or discuss this with your doctor. And be open to counseling. Sometimes it's tough to get out of a depressive slump. It's as if you're in quicksand sinking little by little, but there's nothing you can do about it. Yes, there is—you can seek treatment.

Anxiety

Anxiety may occur in seniors as we face life changes and the stress that comes with them.[7] Multiple stressors occurring at the same time make it hard to deal with the changes. Some risk factors include financial insecurity, the death of a loved one, and loss of independence. Anxiety also has a genetic component and can run in families.[8]

If those feelings of nervousness become overwhelming and limit all that you want to do, it may be a sign of an anxiety disorder. Anxiety symptoms vary from one person to another, but some include the following:[9]

- nervousness
- restlessness
- apprehension
- fear
- panic
- headaches
- worrying
- nausea
- dry mouth
- excessive sweating
- trembling fingers/hands
- cold or sweaty hands
- obsessive thoughts
- overreacting
- racing heart
- decreased memory and focus
- insomnia
- not engaging in routine activities
- fearing the worst in situations
- uncontrollable emotions

When these symptoms cause you to stop engaging in the activities you previously enjoyed, there is a problem. Discuss your symptoms with your health care provider. Usually, the physician rules out potential physical illnesses that may cause the symptoms. If none are found, they may refer you to a counselor, psychologist, or psychiatrist. These professionals use interviews and assessment tools to diagnose the mental health issue.

Many adults do not seek help from a medical professional because they are ashamed. Anxiety disorders are a chronic medical condition that cannot be controlled on your own. These disorders, like depression, are treated with therapy and medication. A counselor can help you identify triggers and learn healthy responses to them.

In addition, the following strategies can help you deal with anxiety:[10]

- exercise and physical activity
- low-carb, healthy diet
- adequate sleep
- meditation
- yoga
- deep breathing
- fewer caffeinated beverages
- avoiding alcohol
- journaling thoughts and feeling
- sharing feelings with loved ones

Refined carbohydrates and high-sugar foods and beverages raise blood-sugar levels. Heightened blood-sugar levels cause the pancreas to release insulin. In turn, blood-sugar levels plummet (reactive hypoglycemia), and you feel wiped out—devoid of energy.[11] The body releases adrenaline to counteract the low blood sugar, and this causes anxiety and even panic attacks.[12] I believe that is why the incidence of anxiety disorders has increased in our society. Blood sugar fluctuations also cause a person to be more irritable and short-tempered.[13] Be sure to reduce your sugar intake to lessen episodes of anxiety.

There are natural products such as kava, cannabidiol (CBD), and medical marijuana that may help with anxiety.[14] They are herbs and plants that may be less invasive to the body than pharmaceutical medications. Ask your physician about these more natural forms of treatment.

Severe anxiety is not a normal part of aging.[15] Today's anxiety treatments are safe and effective, and they can assist you with feeling like your old self again.

Faith

You should pray about when is the best time to retire and be sure to plan for it well in advance. You may want to reduce your work hours over time versus stopping working completely all at once. No matter what, we all die. And we can't take our wealth or material possessions with us. However, God gives the crown of glory to those who love him. James 1:12 says, "God blesses those who patiently endure testing and temptation. Afterward they will receive the crown of life that God has promised to those who love him."

We grow closer to the Lord when we develop spiritual habits. Pray throughout the day, not just before meals or at bedtime. Call upon him when you need help. For example, each morning, say hello to the Lord and ask him to be with you throughout your day. As the day progresses, remain in contact with him spiritually through talking to him and asking for his help as you need it. Nothing is too big or small for you to converse with him about. He wants to be a part of your life. You are not alone. God sees your troubles.

Spend time with God through reading a devotion or a Bible verse, as well as spending meditative time in his presence. Through salvation, we received the Holy Spirit. Receiving God's Spirit is like a seed, which needs spiritual nutrients to grow. As the seed grows, so does our ability to access his power through the Spirit.

Fellowship with other Christians through taking a Bible study, attending Sunday school or a small group, or going to Wednesday evening prayer services. It is through small groups that we get to know others. A Christian community of friends is beneficial anytime in our life, but even more so as we age. How are you socializing with other Christians?

Strengthen your ability to face the challenges of aging through staying close to God. He will see you through this life until you receive the crown of life.

PERSONAL AND PRACTICAL APPLICATION

1. What mental health stressor do you have going on in your life right now? Have you done anything to manage it? What else can you do to find additional support?
2. Have you created a will or an estate yet? If not, what do you plan to do?
3. Do you have a central location for your essential documents (will, birth certificate, Social Security card, passwords, and so on)? Have you informed your family of where these documents are located?
4. Do you need to post a Do Not Resuscitate order for a loved one or yourself?
5. Have you visited a funeral home or mortuary to make your funeral arrangements yet? Have you expressed your wishes to your family about your desired arrangements?
6. If you are currently grieving the loss of a loved one, have you gotten emotional help through counseling or joined a support group?
7. Do you need to declutter your home? What areas do you need to work on first? Who could you ask to assist you with this task?
8. Do you need to make modifications to your home because of an illness or for safety? Do you need to add grab bars to your shower?
9. Do you suffer from symptoms of depression or anxiety? If yes, what have done about it? Is it time to seek help from a health care provider?

CHAPTER 10

CREATED FOR WORK, COMMUNITY, AND BALANCE

Give a man health and a course to steer, and he'll never stop to trouble about whether he's happy or not.
—George Bernard Shaw

We've covered a lot of ground so far in learning to age well and live the lives God created us to experience. We must care for the physical body through diet, exercise, brain and gastrointestinal health, detoxification, and balanced hormones. We gain emotional and mental health through stress management. Now we will explore how God created us to have purpose and to work. But through our multitude of tasks, we need to achieve a balanced life and prioritize self-care. Not enough of either of these will keep us from a sense of fulfillment and extra years of life to enjoy.

THE SECRET TO A SATISFIED LIFE

As people age closer to sixty-five, many thoughts turn to retirement, although paid retirement did not exist in the US prior to the Social Security pension enactment in 1935.[1] Currently, our society portrays retirement as a season for vacation and idleness. Yet in the Bible, people worked throughout their lives. Hard work is a virtue. King Solomon observed that those who were idle were among the least happy. He said in Ecclesiastes 3:22, "So I saw that there is nothing better for a person than to enjoy their work, because that is their lot" (NIV). We are happiest when our days are filled with meaningful, productive labor.

Susan U. Neal

What is the secret to a happy life? To enjoy your work—whatever that may be—employment, a hobby, or volunteering. For many, decades in a chosen career, or in caring for a home and family, brought personal fulfillment. But even in this age of retirement, you can find ways to be productive and not idle. For example, you could volunteer at a pregnancy resource center. While answering calls and talking to distressed young women, you could save life after life. Or you could create a beautiful garden for your family and others to enjoy. My mother did this through her garden club. Whatever activity you choose, find your divine purpose, and let God be your employer. He's the best boss.

How do you ensure you enjoy your labor, whether still employed or after retirement? Use the gifts God gave you. Take a spiritual gifts test to determine your God-given talents. If your work uses those gifts, you will appreciate what you do more because you were created for that purpose. You will wake up excited about the day ahead.

My spiritual gifts are teaching, administration, and hospitality. I love hosting and teaching Bible studies. Leading a study group for twelve years spiritually prepared me to write *Christian Study Guide for 7 Steps to Get Off Sugar and Carbohydrates*. This was my fourth book after starting a new career as a Christian author in my midfifties.

How did I end up being a writer? I sure didn't start in that direction. After visiting a nursing home in high school, I decided to become a nurse so I could help others. I received a bachelor of science degree in nursing, and then worked for two years at UF Health Shands Hospital on a kidney transplant floor. However, this profession was emotionally and physically tough. Dealing daily with death and trauma took its toll on me. To handle the devastating aspects of the job, I hardened my heart. After two years, I chose to change my circumstances. We can't stop getting older, but we can change many aspects of our lives.

If you do not love your work, change it. The years you work are a major portion of your life. Get out of your situation if you hate it. Instead, look for a new job or a hobby you enjoy. Find work that taps into your spiritual gifts, and hopefully it will be in line with God's purpose for you.

After leaving nursing, I took an aptitude test that indicated I would be an excellent administrator in the health care field, especially since I was a registered nurse. My spiritual gift of administration, along with my skills, affected the results of that evaluation.

God divinely created each of us. And we're all different. My sister is artistically talented as a metal sculptor. She represented her state of North Carolina by being invited to the White House to present First Lady Bush with an ornament to be placed on the president's Christmas tree. This tree had ornaments created by artists to represent their states.

I can't create like my sister does. But I have organizational skills God placed within me. When I use those talents, it's like I'm not working at all. In fact, I am filled with joy. When I teach, I get excited and gain energy versus being depleted because I am working out of the strength God gave me. Now I understand why I became the official trainer who oriented all new nursing personnel to the kidney transplant floor. Through the spiritual gift of teaching, I thoroughly enjoyed coaching each new nurse, and my supervisor recognized my natural talent.

After I left my nursing position, I went to graduate school for my master of business administration and master of health science degrees. I landed an internship at Mayo Clinic Jacksonville. At the end of my internship, they offered me a job as the salary administrator and job analyst. I thoroughly enjoyed writing job descriptions for each position at the clinic. I learned all about salaries and raises.

Education should never stop throughout your life. Continued learning helps prevent cognitive decline. Taking in new knowledge happens throughout your employment years but also as you take on new hobbies. You learn something new when starting a new activity, such as knitting, painting, or fishing.

After three years of working at Mayo, I became the administrator of a dozen medical and surgical specialties and managed over a hundred employees. Wow, I never dreamed I would move up into such a high administrative role. But when you use your natural God-given gifts and talents, it shows.

I left my career to become a stay-at-home mom—which is also a job that requires hard work! In fact, I believe raising our children for the Lord is our highest and most difficult job. After twenty years, I felt the divine calling to write. My nursing and health care background matched perfectly with a passion for writing healthy-living books. In my fifties, I followed my God-inspired dream, even though I made Cs in my college writing class. We can learn new things! I feel satisfied helping others improve their health and longevity through this career. Are you satisfied with your current work, hobby, or volunteer role? If not, try something else that taps into your spiritual gifts.

To obtain the full life God wants us to receive, we must make choices and take action. Decide to make the first step to find your divine purpose. Using your time and talents will fulfill you.

COMMUNITY

While our hard work is a virtue and brings satisfaction, it should never be our only desire. We need stimulating work and hobbies but also strong relationships. When we have both, we enjoy a balanced life. God made us to live in community with others, not in isolation. When we are alone, our mental health suffers, and we may become depressed.

When I was married and raising three daughters, we attended a United Methodist Church for twenty years. Through this church I found a delightful Christian community for our entire family. Do you have a church you attend?

Building relationships through a spiritual community requires more than simply attending church, however. Like anything, it takes effort. We need to get involved. At first, I attended a women's Bible study led by the pastor's wife. I was raised in a Catholic home, and we never read the Bible. Our family didn't even own a Bible. This was the first time I had ever attended such a group, and I learned so much.

The Bible study opened a whole new world to me. I learned spiritual wisdom and understanding I never knew before. And I met lifelong friends.

This wonderful community of women provided me with the deep friendships I needed while raising my kids. Many of us had young children, and the church provided a nursery service for free. After Bible study, we always went out to lunch and shared life together.

I also started another small group at our church called the Kids Club. About a dozen families with kids got together for monthly potluck dinners. The kids ran around and played as the parents chatted. Again, this community of friends provided the emotional support we all needed during this season of our lives. Those families are still some of my closest friends.

Unfortunately, after twenty years at this church, the congregation split. A new pastor arrived who gutted the leadership of the church. Half of the members left. It was extremely painful leaving this community of faith. Have you ever experienced a split in a church congregation? I never want to go through such a devastating experience again.

My divorce was like that congregational split. I no longer got together with the same couples we were friends with when married. I had to find new friends.

One Friday night at a local restaurant, I saw a group of women dining, and I knew a couple of them. I spoke with them, and they invited me to join them on Friday nights for dinner. At first, I met them monthly. Now I don't miss a Friday night unless I'm out of town. The new friends provided the emotional support I needed during my divorce. Now at this senior stage of my life (my sixties), they are my closest friends. We support each other through life.

Life has a lot of bumps in the road, so it is vital to have a community to share your closest feelings with. What have you done to meet new friends? In addition to my Friday night dinner group, I joined a book club. Every month, someone chooses a book for the group to read and hosts a dinner at their home for discussion. I've read a delightful assortment of fiction books with this group. Are you in a club or small group? Do you have a local church community? If you can't find one, create one. If you don't like to read, try audiobooks and you can still be involved in a book club.

To meet people with similar interests, become involved in an activity you enjoy. My mother was in garden and bridge clubs. Exercise classes are fun. Most communities have websites to help you locate local groups that share your same passions.

You can also get involved in your community through volunteering. Don't keep your talents, time, and wisdom to yourself. Share them to benefit others. Volunteering deepens your sense of purpose. Look for places or people you can serve. Some examples are Big Brothers Big Sisters, hospitals, hospice, church, or even a family member who needs help. Who has God placed in your path that you can serve? To read more about volunteering, see chapter 8.

I once asked a physician for advice regarding longevity. He shared that his oldest and healthiest patients had a project, people, and purpose. Working on some sort of mission or endeavor gave them resolve. They had individuals in their life that they cared about and who, in turn, cared about them. They focused their attention on people and activities that gave them purpose.

But not everyone has such a mission. Unfortunately, as we age, we may become socially isolated, which negatively affects our well-being. Not having friends or family to call upon can harm our mental health. Risk factors for isolation include these below:[2]

- living alone
- unable to leave home
- being a caregiver
- a major life change (move, death of a spouse, disease)
- lack of a sense of purpose
- feeling disconnected from others

Evaluate your social network and, if needed, act to strengthen the relationships you have and make new ones. Stay in touch with family members and friends through phone calls or online. What can you do to make more connections? Invite someone over for coffee or meet for lunch. Call an old friend to join you for a movie or visit an art museum. Go next door and meet a neighbor. Take a class to learn something new or start a hobby you've always wanted to try. Now is the time, as most of us are less busy than at any other time in our lives.

No matter your age, you need social connection to thrive. Animals can provide a source of comfort too. Recognizing that you have become isolated is the first step toward improving your quality of life. We can't stop the clock of aging, but we can choose to enhance our social network, and that may mean getting out of our comfort zone to make the first move.

BALANCE

We all need balance in our lives—time for exercise, work, and relationships. Incorporating meaningful activities into our routine improves quality of life. We want to manage our limited time and energy productively.

Balance starts with recognizing our unique sense of purpose, an aim that gets us up in the morning with anticipation and vitality. It may be taking care of your grandson, volunteering, or reading a new mystery, or participating in hobbies like golf, singing, or bird-watching. Whatever it is, having a purpose brings contentment.

Another crucial element of a balanced life is good relationships. Stay engaged with family and friends. We need social stimulation and to know that someone cares for us and can lend an ear when we need to share. When we meet others through community involvement, it expands our social lives, and offers an added sense of purpose.

With more time on our hands, too much downtime is an easy path to idleness and lack of movement. We must intentionally maintain physical activity through exercise, sports, or hobbies. If we don't use our muscles, we lose muscle mass and are more susceptible to falls and injury. Even with limited mobility, you may be able to participate in water aerobics or chair yoga. Both are excellent forms of activity. Create new ways to incorporate exercise into your weekly routine.

A primary goal as we age should be to maintain not only a healthy body but also a sharp mind. Mental stimulation is fundamental. What type of activities do you perform that challenge your mind? To review more ideas, see chapter 4.

When we don't manage stress, it can lead to burnout. I tend to overwork and not achieve as much balance as I desire. My inner drive wants to accomplish instead of relaxing. Caregiving, high-stress jobs, and even too many volunteer hours can cause burnout. Unfortunately, we don't always recognize unprocessed, long-term stress. It shows up through fatigue, discontent, dissatisfaction with work, and negative thoughts. This may cause you to become disconnected from family and friends. I've recognized I was suffering from these symptoms several times in my life. I needed to make changes.

To recover from burnout, focus on self-care. During one season of my life, I was so busy working and keeping up household duties, I never slowed down to do my morning devotions. Has your spiritual life suffered because of stressful work or too many activities? Taking time to commune with your Creator is the foundation of a joyful life and will help you keep the other areas in balance.

Self-care also involves scheduling the ways you look after other aspects of your personal life. Don't put yourself last in your priority list, or you won't be able to give out to others. So make time for medical and dental appointments, haircuts, and downtime to relax. Some people relax by shopping, lunching with friends, or reading a book. Be sure enjoyable downtime is part of your self-care balanced routine to avoid burnout.

Time management helps you use your time most efficiently. Some time management strategies include creating to-do lists and prioritizing items, while setting goals for accomplishing them. Group activities together to maximize your time, such as making all your phone calls or checking emails at a certain time. If you take a walk, either outside or inside, while performing some tasks, you'll exercise your body at the same time. Set up your appointments or errands for one day instead of spreading them out over the week. Silence your cell phone when accomplishing a big task to stay focused. These time management techniques help you accomplish more in less time.

Sleep and a healthy diet are vital to a balanced life too. Constructive activities like music, art, and walks in nature ground us. Prayer and scripture meditation anchor us to our Creator. In summary, the components of a balanced life include the following:

- Know your purpose.
- Connect with family and friends.
- Participate in hobbies.
- Volunteer in the community.
- Plan exercise.
- Maintain a healthy body and mind.
- Manage stress.
- Recognize and prevent burnout.
- Manage time effectively.
- Care for yourself.
- Eat a healthy diet.
- Sleep well.
- Connect with God.

MAINTAINING BALANCE

Once we learn to become well balanced, life has a way of throwing us off again. In order to maintain a good level of balance, we need to evaluate what we do and don't do. Saying yes to one activity means saying no to another because we are not as energetic as we once were. It's okay to politely decline. Saying no is how we set boundaries. Learn to listen to your body; if you are tired, rest. If you are too drained after taking care of a grandchild, say no to an evening outing. But make sure that babysitting was your highest priority over the evening event. If not, you may need to say no to babysitting. Understanding our limitations helps us enjoy a more balanced schedule.

I love having a schedule. On Fridays, I teach Christian yoga, work out, run errands, and attend a Bible study. In the evening, I get together with friends for dinner. It's a busy day, but it is part of my weekly schedule that I can count on. We are habitual, and maintaining a routine brings comfort for most of us and helps us maintain a balanced life.

Within that schedule we need to build in time to relax, like enjoying a bubble bath after taking care of a grandchild, which is exhausting. Or maybe we relax by watching a movie. I am enjoying The Chosen series. Each episode brings Jesus's life to light. Try to do something you enjoy every day. Whether it is taking a walk, talking with a friend, or watching a movie.

One constant in our lives is change. We will always encounter it. Having an attitude of accepting change as part of life will enhance our ability to adapt. For example, we may not be able to continue living in the same home without assistance as we age. And we all die one day, even with a heathy life. Accepting this and looking forward to our future eternal life with God will go a long way toward enjoying a satisfied life.

To summarize, the following useful tactics help you maintain balance:

- Learn to say no.
- Set boundaries.
- Listen to your inner voice.
- Prioritize.

- Recognize your limitations.
- Maintain a schedule.
- Take time to relax.
- Keep your spirituality intact.
- Do something you enjoy every day.
- Embrace change instead of resisting it.
- Look forward to your future eternal life with the Lord.

Living a balanced life is hard to achieve. You want to spend time on your projects and hobbies, as well as with family and friends. Figuring out how to do both within the time and energy you have is key. Creating boundaries and evaluating when to say yes are two crucial ways to achieve balance.

We must accept that we will do less than we could accomplish when we were younger. We need feel no shame in losing a few steps. As we age, we don't have as much energy. It is fine to focus on one goal for the day. Prioritize what is most important each day. It takes work to age gracefully. Embrace the wisdom that comes with age. You have more experience and more time to do the things you enjoy now than ever before. Work on achieving your perfect balance.

SELF-CARE PRACTICES

Self-care can mean different things to different people. It is a set of activities we take part in to improve ourselves both internally and externally. We all need to take care of our physical, mental, emotional, and spiritual selves. When we take time to nourish ourselves, we are happier and healthier.

We neglect ourselves for a multitude of reasons. We don't have time; we take care of others; or we simply don't make ourselves a priority. However, we need to prioritize our needs because when we do, our productivity increases. We can promote our own self-care in a variety of ways, but we have to do so intentionally, or other responsibilities will take over.

A large part of self-care is physical. In addition to simple hygiene and a good diet, we have to regularly care for parts of our bodies. Some of these strategies may seem basic, but it's easy to let our personal care slide, especially when our energy levels are lower now.

Regular dental cleanings are not only important to keep your teeth healthy, but they also have been found to prevent dementia. Periodontal disease and bacteria are harmful to our brains.[3] Take care of your teeth and gums through flossing, brushing, and using a water flosser to maintain a healthy smile and mind. I use an app to ensure the toothpaste and mouthwash I buy are nontoxic. We need to be careful what we apply to our skin and gums.

Medical appointments and regular blood tests ensure that our electrolytes, blood cells, and organs function properly. If the tests show we are low in vitamin D or iron, we can take supplements, which ease the symptoms of fatigue associated with these low levels. Routine mammograms and colonoscopies check for cancer. Early diagnosis is lifesaving.

Then our eyes need attention. As we age, most of us need glasses for reading, and many will eventually need surgery for cataracts. We may also be more prone to eye diseases that generally start at an older age. Schedule optical appointments to adjust your lens prescription. See an ophthalmologist for additional eye health. Improved vision enhances our life.

To remain active, we walk a lot, so we must take care of our feet. Proper footwear was discussed in chapter 3. In addition, we should trim our toenails. But getting down to our feet is not always easy. Pedicures and manicures care for our nails, and make you feel splendidly indulgent. My daughters and I enjoy getting a mani and pedi together. It's fun to socialize while being pampered.

I also indulge in chiropractic adjustment and massage several times a year. Adjusting my vertebral column to ensure it is in proper alignment makes my body work better. Working out muscle tension through a massage is therapeutic and detoxifying. Both are valuable.

A new haircut makes me feel pretty. It's amazing to me how nice my hair looks after the hairdresser styles it, as compared to when I try to mimic what she did. I also like to get a facial several times a year, which removes the layer of dead skin and vitalizes my face. Maintain a healthy beauty routine and moisturize your skin daily. I use nontoxic products on my skin, and you can find these within any budget, which will help your skin flourish without toxicity.

Of course, eating a healthy diet of God's food (vegetables, fruits, grains, nuts, seeds, and meat) is part of taking care of our bodies. Hydrate with an adequate amount of clean, filtered water every day.

As part of your weekly routine, find ways to move your body in any fashion you enjoy. And you don't necessarily need a gym membership. Even taking care of a twenty-pound baby is a workout. You lift those twenty pounds in many ways. Read chapter 3 to stimulate your ideas of exercise best suited for you, your lifestyle, and your budget.

Sometimes in life we feel "less than." We look around and see others succeeding where we don't. Don't live an insecure life. Take care of your emotional self by increasing confidence. Speaking positive affirmations to yourself enhances self-esteem. For instance, give yourself a pep talk before performing a challenging task. When I run into a technological issue, I say to myself, *Susan, you can do this. You can do it.* And I proceed. That affirmation helps me work through the tough issue. Intrinsic affirmations are beneficial and make your resolve stronger. You can also find scripture verses that remind you of the truth of how valued and loved you are by God. Find ways to memorize and recite these to yourself when faced with a lack of confidence, or just to start your day on a positive note.

Self-care isn't all done in isolation. A vital part of taking care of ourselves is quality time with family and friends. So is cultivating your relationship with your significant other. Schedule a date night regularly to spend together time. Phone calls and lunch or coffee dates with family or friends fulfill our need for social interaction. Attend weekly church services, fellowship, and small group meetings so you feel part of a spiritual community.

Every day we should incorporate downtime to relax. This gives our bodies and our minds a chance to decompress from the stresses of the day. We can unwind in a variety of ways. Some may enjoy lying in a hammock in the backyard. I enjoy drinking a cup of tea on my back porch listening to the birds in the morning or watching the sunset in the evening. Find a way to relax that you enjoy. We should also honor the Sabbath by resting. This is a hard one for most of us. I've planned plenty of household chores on Sunday. But through a recent Bible study, I learned we should make an appointment time with God. It is a special day to spend time with him—in addition to attending church. From Saturday evening at sunset until Sunday evening at sunset, I try not to check my emails or do other work-related activities. I don't always succeed, but I try.

Schedule vacations, even if only weekend trips. You can choose cost-effective staycations, where you don't have to drive and can learn more about your own hometown. When we are away from the house and all the business of keeping it up, we allow our body, mind, and soul to rest. When we return to our routine, we have more vitality.

God created us to live in nature, yet we rarely put our bare feet on the earth. Grounding or earthing occurs when we take off our shoes and put our feet on the ground. When the body gets in contact with the Earth's natural charge, it stabilizes its physiological makeup.[4] Make it a point to put your feet on nature's ground for a few minutes, several times a week. Also, use your sense of feel to touch a flower petal, leaf, or blade of grass. While you are outside, let your skin soak up the rays of the sun to get some vitamin D naturally.

Our minds need as much self-care attention as our bodies. Engage your brain in mental stimulation as much as possible. Learn more about an interesting topic. I've always wanted to know more about the constellations. Listen to a podcast or read a book. Some apps have mental exercises to stimulate your mind for a few minutes at a time. You could learn another language or a new hobby, basically anything that interests you and you find mentally invigorating.

Engage in activities that bring you fulfillment. For example, after my brother-in-law retired, he joined a group of volunteers who maintain the Appalachian Trail in North Carolina. The men gather their equipment, drive to a trailhead, and walk for miles cutting fallen trees and encroaching vegetation along the trail. They get great physical exercise, socialize with each other, and feel satisfaction from a job well done. They know what they are doing allows thousands of visitors to hike through God's glorious mountains.

You can feel a sense of pleasure through any hobby. Whether it is knitting socks or growing vegetables. One friend of mine has an eighty-six-year-old mother who—even with failing eyesight—creates "fidget quilts" for autistic children and adults in long-term care facilities. She gets to stimulate her mental creativity and engage her imagination. She meets weekly with other women on these projects, which enhances her relationships. And this activity gives her a sense of purpose.

We also need spiritual contentment through spending time with our Creator. This may include reading the Bible or meditating with the Lord. Jesus said, "I am leaving you with a gift—peace of mind and heart. And the peace I give is a gift the world cannot give" (John 14:27). We cannot be truly fulfilled or obtain peace without connecting spiritually to God.

Don't neglect your emotional side. We find emotional nourishment through laughter, practicing gratitude, writing positive affirmations, and journaling our thoughts and feelings. When we focus on positivity and uplifting self-talk, we nourish the soul. Seek ways you can perform acts of kindness in your day. It will make someone's day and make you feel good intrinsically. Enjoy beauty in your day. Something as simple as looking at fresh flowers on the dining room table improves our emotional outlook.

We all have an artistic side. God made us in his image. God is a creator, and we are too. We love to create, whether it is a delicious meal or a painted masterpiece. Yet we are prone to neglect this part of ourselves. We feel as though it is not as significant as our work or service. But holistically, it is. Get in touch with your creative self. Try painting, drawing, or gardening. Write a poem. Take some great photos. Dance. Listen to music. Do whatever helps you connect to this God-given part of you.

Last, but definitely not least, we need to sleep well. We should stay in bed at least eight hours. Even resting the body without fully engaging in sleep is beneficial. I have a bottle of magnesium at my bedside that I take before lying down. This mineral helps the muscles relax.[5] I don't drink caffeine after two p.m. If I do, I will not be able to fall asleep quickly. Physical activity ensures I sleep soundly, as my body is tired.

Which of these self-care practices are you using, and which can you begin to insert into your life?

- regular dental, medical, and optical appointments
- mammograms and colonoscopies
- pedicures and manicures
- chiropractic adjustments and massages
- hair appointments
- facials
- healthy diet and hydration
- exercise
- social interaction
- spiritual fellowship
- relaxing downtime
- vacations
- grounding
- sunshine
- mental stimulation
- activities that provide fulfillment
- hobbies
- spiritual nourishment
- emotional sustenance
- artistic outlets
- sleeping well

We should also decrease or remove unhealthy habits such as smoking cigarettes, eating high-sugar desserts, and drinking alcoholic beverages in excess. Try to replace a negative habit with a self-care practice instead.

We all need to prioritize ourselves by scheduling "me" time. Look at the list above and determine what you currently do. What tactics should you add to your routine? You could ask yourself what activities bring joy, peace, fulfillment, or energy. Write down the practices you want to incorporate into your life. Schedule them on your calendar.

This year, after I analyzed what I did and did not do, I created a monthly checklist divided by four weeks. On the left side of the page, I listed all the self-care items I wanted to ensure I perform at least weekly. For example, I want to walk two miles, read my Bible study, and connect socially a couple times a week. I also added to my list a negative habit that I don't want to partake in excessively, so I document how often I do it (like eating desserts or scrolling too much on social media). Monitoring helps me recognize when it is excessive. Each day, I check an item or two off my weekly list. At the end of a week or month, I can see what I am lacking and need to work on. These habits improve my well-being holistically. When you prioritize taking care of yourself, both you and the people in your life benefit.

Share your self-care plan with a family member or friend. Don't keep your goals or the why behind your goals a secret. Tell others. This is the major difference between those who succeed in meeting their goals and those who do not.

For example, if you want to walk ten miles each week, tell others you are going to do this. Send them a text with a screenshot of your number of miles walked at the end of each week. You affirm to yourself and others that you will accomplish this task. When we verbalize something, it becomes more real to us. Declare what you want to accomplish, why you want to accomplish it, and how you're going to attain it. This makes it more likely to happen.

God intended for us to work. Working for money or volunteering brings intrinsic satisfaction. Choose how and on what you will devote your time, even if it is a delightful hobby. Socialize with family, friends, or members of your community. God did not intend for us to live in isolation. Gain balance by managing all your activities. Make self-care a priority. You and everyone around you will benefit when you do. Take a holistic approach to living your best life.

PERSONAL AND PRACTICAL APPLICATION

1. Do you have the support of close friends? Who can you call to share your burdens and blessings with?
2. Have you ever moved or experienced a situation where you had to develop new friendships? What did you do to meet new friends? What can you do now to make more connections?
3. What type of activities do you perform that challenge your mind? Do you read, put together puzzles, or play word games on your phone? What new mental stimulation will you try?
4. What hobby have you always wanted to try? What is stopping you from pursuing it?
5. Do you fill your idle time with activities that fulfill you? What do you enjoy most?
6. Do you have an eternal purpose? If not, what can you do to find it?

7. Do you suffer from symptoms of burnout? What steps can you take to heal from it?
8. Do you arrange regular dental, medical, and optical appointments as needed? Which one do you need to schedule? Take care of that appointment today.
9. Evaluate the list of self-care strategies. Which ones are you doing? Which ones do you need to incorporate into your life?

CHAPTER 11

CULTIVATE YOUR SPIRITUAL HEALTH

Look to your health; and if you have it, praise God, and value it next to a good conscience; for health is the second blessing that we mortals are capable of; a blessing that money cannot buy.

—Izaak Walton

The human spirit cannot be separated on this earth from the mind and body. Our spiritual self is as much a part of us as our physical, mental, and emotional facets. When all are in alignment, we have the greatest opportunity for a healthy, long life.

We've discussed how our spiritual lives intersect with our other areas of life. For example, we open up our social and emotional selves when we help others and give back to our community through volunteer work and ministry. Incorporating gratitude into our lives is a way to focus outside ourselves when dealing with difficult issues or poor health. And listening to and singing praise music lifts one's mood. Now let's go deeper into understanding how our spiritual side contributes to a healthier, longer life.

SPIRITUAL JOURNEY

In this life, we are on a spiritual journey. God formed Adam from the earth. When we die, our bodies return to dust, but our spirits go back to God, as indicated in Ecclesiastes 12:7: "And the dust returns to the ground it came from, and the spirit returns to God who gave it" (NIV).

Before we were born, our spirits were in paradise with God, bathed in his presence. There were no challenges, no opportunities to choose between right and wrong, nor to learn selflessness. When our spirit entered this world at birth, in an earthly body, we got the opportunity to grow, develop, and mature as a human being.

Unfortunately, during our life on earth, we can't remember that our spirits were with God before we were born. Only a relationship with God can satiate the longing in our hearts. Many do not recognize where this longing comes from—missing our Lord's presence. Instead, we turn to worldly delights that do not satisfy our souls because only God can.

We fall into sin and become filthy from it. The greatest consequence of sin is eternal separation from God. Unfortunately, we can't be close to God when we lead a sinful life. But once we ask for forgiveness, God chooses not to remember our sins. In Isaiah 43:25, God explains, "I—yes, I alone—will blot out your sins for my own sake and will never think of them again." So once we recognize our sins and repent (including turning away from the sins and turning toward God), he chooses not to remember our sins anymore.

I found the following revelations about prayer. Psalm 66:18 tells us, "If I had not confessed the sin in my heart, the Lord would not have listened." If we have a sinful heart, God won't listen to our prayers. So when I sit down to pray, I assess my heart and ask God to point out anything sinful. Then I ask for his forgiveness.

Amazingly, God chooses not to remember our sins once we have confessed with a sincere heart. But we must learn to forgive ourselves. God loves us and wants us to spend eternity with him. God provided a means for us to live forever in his presence, through our belief in Jesus. God's followers gain eternal life through Jesus Christ's death and acknowledging Jesus as our savior, which fulfills our lifelong search. No price was too high for God to have our spirits return to him—their ultimate home. God gave us the gift of the resurrection of the dead.

But God does not want the sinful, broken version of you in eternity. Psalm 139 tells us he knew us before we were formed in our mother's womb. He loves you and hates the suffering you've endured in this life.

Yet God can erase the trauma of this world and transform you into the ideal version of you—no matter how low you have sunk in this fallen world. He does this only when you give him control of your life. Ask for his will to be done in your life, not your own. The only way out of this painful world and into paradise is through a new path, following Jesus and with God as our focus.

HOLY SPIRIT'S GUIDANCE

I remember the first time I recognized the Holy Spirit's leading in my life. I was in my thirties and had recently rededicated to my life to Christ and was baptized. While planting flowers in my garden, I felt an inner voice telling me to plant the seedling in a specific spot. I refused to obey. A few days later, the plant died.

Shortly thereafter, as I got ready to go to church for a Saturday workday, I felt the inner voice tell me to bring an extra hat. *That's ridiculous,* I thought. But I listened this time since the plant died. When I arrived at church, I asked a friend walking to his car, "Why are you leaving?"

"Because I forgot my hat. I have to go back home and get one to cover my bald head."

"I brought an extra hat. It must be for you."

After that, I recognized the Holy Spirit's quiet voice within me. I came to realize that the Spirit's influence was like what I was taught in college about your conscience. I feel the Spirit leading me with simple things in life.

Have you ever looked for something in your house you can't find? When this happens, I pray. After I pray, I will either come across the item, remember where I put it, or feel the Holy Spirit's urging about where the item is located. Have you ever experienced this phenomenon?

NATURE

Consider nature as a canvas. It contains beautiful colors, textures, and sounds. Being in nature not only brings us emotional and physical health but is restful for our soul and spirit. Bathe in it daily. Do not stay indoors all the time.

God's canvas changes seasonally with the colors of the leaves and petals of the flowers. In spring, the leaves of many trees are a brilliant lime green, and the redbud, tulip trees, and azaleas burst with colorful blooms. In the summer, the leaves thicken and darken, and many other flowers grace the landscape. In the fall, the color of the leaves is magnificent—gold, yellow, and red. Many leaves disappear in the winter, and the trees are stark—kind of like the thirst in our soul for connecting with the Lord spiritually. But the entire process is rebirthed in the spring so we may enjoy its breathtaking glory. If I lived one hundred years, I wouldn't have enough springs to view.

Early in the morning, God's birds sing to us. Open the window and listen to them. Or better yet, sit outside while you spend time with the Lord. Birds sing more in the early morning because the moist air from dew carries their voices farther. God provides dew daily for his animals and insects.

Be like a kid again and look up in the sky at the white, fluffy clouds against the blue canvas. What creations can you see—a fish, dolphin, or horse. Let your imagination go. Rest and relax while enjoying God's splendor.

Sometimes when I am outside, I feel like I should stop what I am doing and look at a bird squawking overhead or touch the petal of a flower. I've learned to listen to this inner voice so I can revel in God's glorious creation. God created nature for us to enjoy. Spend a few moments outside listening to the birds, watching the squirrels, and feeling the breeze. Connect with the Lord who created the world and everything in it. Realign your spirit with his.

Have you ever marveled at the stars in the sky? Sit outside and watch the evening sky. At first, you'll see no stars; then a few appear in the night sky. After a while, stars light up all over. Did you know stars are in the sky during the daytime? But you can't see them until the sunlight diminishes. What an interesting revelation to ponder. Similarly, the Holy Spirit is always with us, but we do not always feel his presence.

Take moments in your life to ponder and delight in God's handiwork that he made for you. Walk or bike in your neighborhood or a nearby park. Sit outside for morning prayer time with God, taking in his creation. You can even notice the beauty of his world as you drive to work or run errands. It's all around you. Don't miss it. Yet as magnificent as nature is, you are God's masterpiece, for he made you in his image. God delights in you (Isaiah 62:4). God created you for a purpose. Have you found your purpose that fulfills an eternal perspective? Seek and find his purpose for you.

Even in your work, you can find God. When you work as unto God, you can look for him in those who cross your path. Work is no longer mundane. No matter what you're doing, or where, your work becomes a ministry where you are the hands and feet of Jesus. Whatever God has called you to do, step out in faith and fulfill that calling. Once you do, your heart will blossom.

DAILY DEVOTIONAL TIME

God puts a longing in our heart to connect with him. Until we do, something is missing in our lives. Jesus said, "I am the bread of life. Whoever comes to me will never go hungry, and whoever believes in me will never be thirsty" (John 6:35 NIV). Quench that thirst by spending a few minutes of your day with the Lord. Besides this devoted time, talk with him throughout the day. He is only a thought away, willing and ready to be a part of your life. He is simply waiting for you to choose him. Have faith that he is with you and will always ensure your needs are met. Believe.

Early in my spiritual journey, I read these two verses:

> Then Jesus said, "Let's go off by ourselves to a quiet place and rest awhile." (Mark 6:31)

> Give all your worries and cares to God, for he cares about you. (1 Peter 5:7)

After reading these verses, I was determined to spend time with the Lord every day. Jesus modeled how to pray in Mark 1:35. "Before daybreak the next morning, Jesus got up and went out to an isolated place to pray."

Prayer was how Jesus connected with God while he was on this earth. If Jesus needed to spend time with God to refuel his spiritual

Cultivate Your Spiritual Health

tank, what does that say for us? We need to spend time with God and enjoy his presence to rejuvenate ourselves each day. We should try to spend a few minutes with the Lord each morning, even if it is simply talking to him as you drive to work.

I feel better when I give my worries to God. I need spiritual restoration that only he can provide. I set up my day with a positive mental attitude by having a cup of Earl Grey tea with the Lord. I sit outside, if weather permits, with a devotional book. After reading the devotion and the scripture for that day, I meditate with the Lord for about five-to-ten minutes by closing my eyes and focusing on my breath. This is when God has an opportunity to penetrate my busy mind.

I can be so active with my daily tasks and thoughts turning in my mind that it never shuts off. It is hard to go to sleep when my mind swirls with contemplations about my long to-do list. That's why each morning, even if it's just for a couple of minutes, I turn my mind off and open it for the Lord to infiltrate. This is when he gives me insights and tasks to do that I would not have thought of on my own.

During my meditation time with the Lord, I'll have thoughts like I should call Heather and check up on her since she was diagnosed with COVID. Or I need to send Lynda a card. I haven't spoken to her in months. Usually, I'm too busy to consider other people's needs versus my own. But God does. He helps me remember to minister to others.

Why don't you try meditating with the Lord? Sit outside and spend time with him as you read your devotion or Bible. At the end, meditate in his presence. Get in a comfortable position, close your eyes, and focus on your breath. Breathe deeply. Try not to think about anything and stay in that position until you feel ready to open your eyes.

I keep a notepad and pen close by so I can jot down his divine thoughts that enter my mind during this time. I call these ideas downloads from the Lord. These downloads help me be a better, happier person.

A couple of days a week, I schedule exercise after my devotional time. I prefer walking two miles or swimming in my pool. Afterward, I blast praise music and sing as I shower and get ready for my day. I let the worship music take over as I sing loudly and passionately to the Lord. I believe singing activates a spiritual energy source within us we don't understand. Singing gives me energy, vitality, and a positive attitude. Next, I break my fifteen-hour fast from dinner the previous night and eat breakfast. Now that is the perfect way to start my day with God at the center of my life. Taking care of my temple brings glory to the Lord.

COMPONENTS OF A SPIRITUAL LIFE

Praying throughout the day, not just at bedtime or before meals, helps you grow closer to the Lord. Pray before you get out of bed each morning and ask the Lord to be with you throughout your day. Remain in contact with him by talking to him and asking for guidance as needed. Nothing is too small for you to converse about with him. God wants to be a part of your life. All you need to do is spiritually connect.

Through salvation, you receive the Holy Spirit. To accept Jesus as your Savior, you need to ask God to forgive you for your sins, tell him you will turn away from those sins, and understand that Jesus died on a cross to pay for everyone's sins. At the moment you ask Jesus to come into your heart and lead your life, you receive the Holy Spirit. Finally, you cast away the sin that has entangled you in this life. You become renewed, a new spiritually alive being who has put on a new nature as described in Colossians 3:8–10. "But now is the time to get rid of anger, rage, malicious behavior, slander, and dirty language. Don't lie to each other, for you have stripped off your old sinful nature and all its wicked deeds. Put on your new nature, and be renewed as you learn to know your Creator and become like him." God's Spirit actually takes up residence within the realm of your mind.

Invite Jesus to be your companion. God is always present and listening to you. The Lord promised that when we walk faithfully with him and he becomes an integral part of our lives, his Spirit will guide us. God desires to gently guide us so we are blessed, and he is glorified.

When we accept Christ as our Savior, God adopts us as his children and loves us unconditionally like a parent. Nothing can take his love away from us. Since we are his children, we can access his power by faith and apply it to any area in our lives.

Receiving God's Spirit is like a seed, which needs to grow. As it grows, so does our ability to access his power through the Holy Spirit.

Cultivate Your Spiritual Health

The following four habits can help you commit yourself to the Lord and live a spiritually healthy life:

1. Submit control of your life to Jesus by asking him to lead your life. Ask him for guidance in all your decisions. Pray for God's will in all the choices you make.
2. Study and memorize scripture verses. When you do, you will place God's values in your heart for leading your life. If you live by what the Bible teaches, you will have a better life. God's Word offers guidance to every area of life, including our health and emotions. You can tap into God's power through reciting Bible verses. As I've indicated previously, speak a verse out loud and with authority, believing in its power. When you memorize scripture, you can unsheathe the sword of the Spirit and slash the Enemy when he tempts. God's Word is an incredible offensive weapon against the voices in our head. What Bible verse do you want to memorize?
3. Spend time with the Lord. I spend time with God each morning with a devotional reading and a cup of tea. Are you spending time with God daily?
4. Fellowship with other Christians is vital. We can do this through participating in a Bible study, attending a small group, or going to Wednesday evening prayer services. Are you socializing with other Christians? Are you attending church? If you are not fellowshipping, how do you plan to incorporate this into your life?

After my divorce, I felt led to find a new church home. It was difficult. But I tried to make it a fun experience. Over a few months, I visited six church services. I rated each one based on the music, friendliness of the members, and content and clarity of the sermon. I stayed at one church for several months because the sermons were spiritually deep. But I lacked connection with others because I did not join any small groups.

Ultimately, I attended another church where I had known some members for more than twenty years. A group from my previous church split attended here, and I felt a deep connection with many of them. But I did not know the majority of the congregation, so I participated in church activities to meet others. I attended occasional luncheons after church and joined a Bible study and a table-talk group. If I had not participated in these events, I wouldn't have met more people than the handful I already knew. Now I thoroughly enjoy attending my church on Sundays. I walk away with a connection with others and a boost in my spirit. As seniors, we are more likely to become isolated. Attending church can help alleviate loneliness.

God's Word can help with stressful situations. When I had an MRI at Mayo Clinic, I got claustrophobic. When you're inside a tube that's only two inches above your nose, it's pretty confining. The anxiety got to me. My heart pounded as I sweated. I had difficulty breathing and staying in the tube. So I began repeating the Bible verse "God is our refuge and strength, an ever-present help in trouble" until the procedure was over (Psalm 46:1 NIV). With God's help, I made it. This is one example of how God's Word helped me deal with a difficult situation.

These faith practices help us stand spiritually strong. Fill your mind, heart, and body with the Spirit of God by putting the right things in your spirit. Is your heart fully committed to God? If yes, how is this demonstrated in your life? If no, what steps will you take to fully commit yourself to him?

FAITH AND PRAYER

Do your prayers focus on God's kingdom and God's will? In the Garden of Gethsemane, Jesus prayed, "My Father! If it is possible, let this cup of suffering be taken away from me. Yet I want your will to be done, not mine" (Matthew 26:39). Prayer is the link between God's will and our work on earth. That is why Jesus got up early and spent time with his Father. We should too.

For example, when Peter was about to be tempted by Satan, what did Jesus do? "I have pleaded in prayer for you, Simon, that your faith should not fail. So when you have repented and turned to me again, strengthen your brothers" (Luke 22:32). Jesus prayed!

I believe prayer is more important than we realize, for it enters the unseen spiritual realm. We should pray more. I wish I did. Here are a few more verses about prayer:

> Are any of you suffering hardships? You should pray. Are any of you happy? You should sing praises. (James 5:13)
>
> The earnest prayer of a righteous person has great power and produces wonderful results. (James 5:16)

Jesus taught us to pray with faith.

SEEK WISDOM, UNDERSTANDING, AND KNOWLEDGE

Genesis 1:27 states, "So God created human beings in his own image." We were made to become more and more like him. When we accept Christ as our Savior, the Holy Spirit takes up residence within us. We experience this divine presence through our minds and thoughts. When we seek God's wisdom, understanding, and knowledge, we experience more of the qualities and expression of the Holy Spirit in our lives. When the human spirit is in communion with God's Spirit, it transcends the physicality of the body. You experience spiritual revelation at a level that is difficult to explain in words.

Wisdom refers to moral reasoning, which begins with the fear of the Lord. God punishes sin and rewards righteousness. Understanding provides the ability to distinguish between good and evil—what is right and wrong. When we experience a personal relationship with God, he reveals spiritual knowledge to us—divine knowledge that is imparted by God.

When the Holy Spirit instructs us through our minds, we discern God's thoughts. First Corinthians 2:11–12 explains this concept: "For who knows a person's thoughts except their own spirit within them? In the same way no one knows the thoughts of God except the Spirit of God. What we have received is not the spirit of the world, but the Spirit who is from God, so that we may understand what God has freely given us" (NIV).

Isn't it amazing to think we actually have the mind of Christ? "For, 'Who can know the Lord's thoughts? Who knows enough to teach him?' But we understand these things, for we have the mind of Christ" (1 Corinthians 2:16). A Spirit-filled person connects the Word of God to their life. Therefore, it is vital that we study the Bible. Understanding God's Word cultivates wisdom, understanding, and knowledge.

God wants to dwell within us through his Spirit. During our life's journey, we need to elevate our physical body into a spiritual being in communion with our Creator. When we do, we obtain fulfillment. Living a full spiritual life, and following God's purpose and meaning for us, leads to a longer and healthier life. How can you seek a deeper relationship with the Lord?

SUMMARY

When we die, what can we take with us? We enter the world naked and leave the same way. However, we do take our good deeds, generosity to those less fortunate, and investments into the kingdom of God. These are our treasures in heaven, along with God's presence.

According to many with near-death experiences, they see their entire life played out before them. Amazingly, they see things not only through their own viewpoint but from the perspectives of those they interacted with on earth. They feel how their choices impacted others. They finally understand the effects of their good deeds and bad ones.

We don't have to almost die in order to see the world with a new perspective. Take time to review your spiritual life through the lens of God's kingdom, and how he would have you see others and yourself. Through this life review, we can finally make sense of this sorrowful world and our strange journey in it. If we labor toward godliness in this lifetime, at the end of our life, we will have a harvest. The harvest includes our experiences, life lessons, good deeds, relationships, and love. As we die, we will review all these memories, both good and bad. Then we arrive in paradise with God or gehenna (hell). If we arrive in paradise, we are finally back home—we passed the test of choosing to follow God in this life. If we do not, we understand why. Examine your heart, if you haven't yet chosen God, and see what is keeping you from following the one who created you and established you for your unique journey and purpose.

PERSONAL AND PRACTICAL APPLICATION

1. Have you found your purpose that fulfills an eternal perspective? How can you seek God's purpose in your life?
2. Have you ever marveled at God's glory through nature? Do you spend time outside? If not, how can you increase your time in nature?
3. Are you spending time with God daily? How can you rejuvenate yourself with God's presence?
4. Have you tried meditating with the Lord? Get in a comfortable position, close your eyes, and focus on your breath. Breathe deeply. Try not to think about anything and stay in that position until you feel ready to open your eyes. What divine wisdom did you receive?
5. Do you socialize with other Christians? If you are not fellowshipping, how do you plan to incorporate this into your life?
6. Have you thought about taking a Bible study, attending a small group, or going to Wednesday evening prayer services? What steps can you take to deepen your Christian walk?
7. What Bible verse do you want to memorize? Write it on an index card and post it visibly in your home so you can memorize it.
8. Is your heart fully committed to God? If yes, how is this demonstrated in your life? If no, what steps will you take to fully commit yourself to him?
9. Do your prayers focus on God's kingdom and God's will? Write a prayer that puts God and his kingdom first and seek to pray it daily.
10. Have you felt communion with God's Spirit? If yes, have you found the experience difficult to explain?
11. When we die, what can we take with us? We take our good deeds, generosity to those less fortunate, and investments into the kingdom of God. What are your treasures in heaven?

CHAPTER 12
HEALTHY HABITS FOR A LONG LIFE

I think a hero is an ordinary individual who finds strength to persevere and endure in spite of overwhelming obstacles.
—Christopher Reeve

If change were easy, we would all effortlessly implement the improvements from this book. But change is not simple. How many times have you tried to set positive lifestyle practices only to be derailed by your own thoughts or life's priorities? You start strong, but your desire fades, and then your willpower. In this chapter, we will dig deep into the psychology of change so you can succeed.

Humans naturally desire comfort, and therefore, follow the path of least resistance. It's a lot nicer to stay indoors than take a long walk in the summer heat or winter cold. It is easier to give up and resign ourselves to mediocre health. Despite our sincere desire to sustain healthy choices, we often fail at maintaining positive change.

Do you feel you can't dig out of your unhealthy situation? Are you stuck? Often, we contribute to our own demise by returning to detrimental behaviors. As Paul wrote in Romans 7:15, "I do not understand what I do. For what I want to do I do not do, but what I hate I do" (NIV). We are not alone.

The first step to creating a consistent and healthy lifestyle is to recognize what trips you up, and what keeps you from the best choices for your body. Keeping track of your patterns will help you honestly evaluate the changes you need. What negative habits do you turn to when you are anxious, stressed, or angry? Write them down. What triggers your negative response? Track your triggers in my book *Healthy Living Journal: Track Your Healthy Eating and Living Habits for Improved Health and Well-Being*. Determine what initiates your unwanted behaviors.

When did a negative habit originate? Write it down. How many toxic habits do you engage in? Try to remember when each began in your life and why. Was it in childhood, after a traumatic event, or after you believed a lie someone told you about yourself? Work on changing one undesirable behavior at a time.

Journal to figure out the reason you act the way you do and why you may struggle to make positive lifelong lifestyle changes. Every time you feel a toxic behavior begin, analyze your thoughts. Where is your undesirable response coming from and how you can stop it? Use the perspective of an objective bystander if you have difficulty understanding your own responses. This type of accountability can help you move forward, as we sometimes have trouble being honest with ourselves.

Once you understand your underlying reasonings and motives, determine an alternate behavior you could employ instead. Consider each of the behaviors you identified. How can you prevent a negative response? Evaluate your answers in your journal so you can create a plan.

Recently, I made a healthy living chart that included my positive and negative habits. Each week, I record how often I engage in these routines. For example, drinking alcohol is a habit I want to decrease, so I document how many days a week I drink. Two days is better than five. I analyze why I want to drink—to decrease my stress. I've learned to tell myself: *I feel great just the way I am. If I drink, my motivation will decrease. I don't need this vice. God fulfills all my needs.* My self-talk helps me decrease this unwanted behavior.

NEGATIVE SELF-TALK

All of us hear negative voices inside our heads. That's right, you are not alone. These voices make compelling arguments to take the easier path for most situations in life. They make excuses and exceptions to dissuade us from doing anything difficult. When we listen to their advice, we sabotage our efforts to make positive change.

The lazy inclination of our mind is not necessarily motivated by evil. It's more about self-preservation. However, King Solomon warns against being lazy in Proverbs 18:9: "A lazy person is as bad as someone who destroys things" and Proverbs 6:10–11:

> A little sleep, a little slumber,
> a little folding of the hands to rest—
> and poverty will come on you like a thief
> and scarcity like an armed man. (NIV)

Our thoughts discourage us from accepting challenges and prevent us from modifying undesirable habits.

The negative voices make us believe we are helpless victims of life's circumstances and are incapable of improving. We lose the battle in our minds before the war for our health begins. Verbalizing pessimistic predictions about what will happen to us in the future leads to self-defeat.

We become our own worst enemy. Fear and self-criticism hold us back. When we listen to the negative voices in our heads, progress stalls. The only way to succeed is to kick the voices out of our minds. Decide to stop listening to the voices' excuses and renew your mind.

We can't achieve perfection in our diet or healthy habits. Instead, we should strive for an improvement over what we have been doing. Don't allow the suggestions in this book to overwhelm you. Embrace what you can do and do not strive for flawlessness because it is unobtainable.

RENEWING THE MIND

You can retrain your brain no matter your beliefs, past trauma, or background because of your brain's neuroplasticity. This term refers to the brain's ability to change when you rewire it to function in a new, different way.[1] Yes, you can train your brain to think differently. You do not have to stay stuck. You can change through shifting the direction of your thoughts.

Second Corinthians 10:5 teaches us how: "We demolish arguments and every pretension that sets itself up against the knowledge of God, and we take captive every thought to make it obedient to Christ" (NIV). We can change the direction of our lives through daily observance of our thoughts and practice, taking every thought captive. Most of us do not think about what is going through our minds. Therefore, we need to assess our thoughts daily and determine why we are feeling or thinking negatively. Awareness is key.

You can control your thoughts—imprison a thought, observe it, and determine whether it is a lie or negative. If it is a lie, figure out the truth. If it is negative, ask God to remove the pessimism from your head. Yet removal is only part of the solution. You must replace what you removed with a positive truth. Find a Bible verse to refute any repeating negative thoughts. Speak that verse out loud when the thought enters your mind. It will surprise you how quickly the falsehood goes away. Write 2 Corinthians 10:5 on an index card and post it somewhere in your home so you can easily recite it.

After doing this analysis every day with every unwanted random thought, your thinking begins to shift. This habit promotes positivity and deters lies. It takes time to retrain your mind, so be persistent.

The more aware you are of your thoughts, the easier it is to recognize what is causing your toxic habits. Identify what drives the thoughts and behaviors that keep you stuck. Once you assess them, you come to recognize you have more control over what is going through your mind than you realized. To renew your mindset, you should work out your mind just like you do your muscles. Replacing negative thoughts with positive ones is a daily practice—twenty-four hours a day, seven days a week—which takes effort and time.

The bumps of life will derail you, but you must continue to slay unwanted thoughts. Be patient. After a while, monitoring your thinking becomes a habit, and the nagging, negative voices no longer plague you. Yes, you can kick those guys out of your life. I know you can because I did.

You can learn not to automatically accept every thought you have as truth. After a while, you believe those lies others told you in the past, which damage your self-worth. The lies cause you to believe less about yourself. You think you are not good enough, and those thoughts limit you from reaching your true potential, the person God knows you can become. The negative voices in your head keep repeating those slanderous words, which develop negative patterns of behavior.

Whether you were told lies about yourself from your parent, spouse, or another voice in your mind—reject them. I created a truth-versus-lie sheet during my divorce. I struggled during that time with negative beliefs about my sense of failure and low self-worth. To fight back and begin to replace negative thoughts, I wrote the slander that had been told to me many times. Beside each lie, I wrote the truth. As I focused on the reality, I expelled those untruthful insults from my mind. I also shared those falsehoods with trusted friends who verified that they were not true.

It is sad and startling that we believe lies about ourselves. These untruths assassinate our character and adversely affect our behavior. Take some time to write the defamations you have believed in your life and dispel them with the truth: God loves you. You are a child of the King of the Universe. You deserve dignity and respect, not slander.

Once we reject the lies, kick the negative voices out of our minds, and notice each thought (especially if it is negative), we make better decisions. Through assessing our thinking, we become more intelligent emotionally. Emotions and thoughts no longer rule us or keep us stuck in unhealthy habits. We learn to change the direction of our thoughts instantly by taking them captive to Jesus Christ.

Ultimately, we replace undesirable thoughts with true and desirable ones. Paul instructs us in Philippians 4:8: "Fix your thoughts on what is true, and honorable, and right, and pure, and lovely, and admirable. Think about things that are excellent and worthy of praise."

Forgiving those who told us lies and harmed us is vital to healthy thinking. We will never completely heal or stop our toxic habits until we do. When we choose to forgive, this act releases us from the grip our perpetrator still has on us. Until we forgive, they still have their talons in our heart. Forgiveness is part of the healing process. You also need to forgive and stop criticizing yourself. Once you do, you're more likely to be successful in improving your lifestyle. Make the choice to forgive. If you can't, ask God to help you. He will.

You can read more about forgiveness in Chapter 8. I used the role-play technique described there to forgive my father. I pretended to sit with my deceased father and explain to him my feelings about an episode in my childhood that had a long-lasting effect on the negative voices in my head. Each evening my father took all his kids to swim at our neighbor's pond. We would pile into the back of his El Camino. One evening, I accidentally sat on the vehicle's antenna, and it broke. In my father's rage, he picked up the antenna and whipped me with it. Welts swelled up on my legs as I ran into the house screaming.

In my forgiveness exercise, I told my father how it felt to be whipped for accidentally breaking the antenna and how wrong it was for him to hit me like that. I did not intentionally break his antenna. Yes, he had previously warned us kids to be careful of it; but I was four years old, and I made a mistake. I cried as I explained that his inappropriate discipline created a rift in our relationship. It was difficult, but through my tears, I told him I forgave him. Peace filled my heart because my wound healed; forgiveness set me free. This intentional action switched my mindset from a fearful child to an adult.

ROOT PROBLEM

Have you realized that the way you are living is not serving you well? Unfortunately, you can't move forward until you acknowledge you have a problem and then figure out the reason. For example, until alcoholics admit their addiction, they can't work to overcome it.

Most of us would rather deny we have an issue. Others don't realize a problem exists. We need to determine why we have a mindset problem—an established attitude we can't seem to change. Was it from the way we were raised? Do we have unhealed wounds from past trauma? Do we need to forgive? Have we ignored the hurt for so long that we have difficulty feeling our genuine emotions? Dig deep and journal the answers to these questions. If you need help in working through these issues, I encourage you to find an accountability or prayer partner or even a professional counselor.

Once we realize a root issue, we can work through it to heal. Otherwise, our life does not improve. We start to change, but ultimately return to our negative habits. Many of us remain in denial of our deep-rooted problems, so nothing improves in our lives. We bury the issue and pretend it doesn't exist. Unless you understand what is holding you back, you can't change. If you can't get unstuck on your own, it may be time to get counseling or hire a life coach.

Journaling is a crucial part of changing behavior. When you write down your thoughts, you can more clearly identify the relationship between your emotional wounds, heart, and brain. Understanding your issue and healing from the root cause helps break the cycle of undesirable habits. This deep inner work is the most important thing you can do because knowing what is holding you back helps you get unstuck.

Replace those bitter roots with self-love. Move from being a victim of your circumstances to realizing you are in control of your own choices. Then you'll discover freedom. You can build a better future and improve your well-being. Believe Philippians 4:13: "I can do all this through him who gives me strength" (NIV).

Document your thoughts and issues in your journal. Identify undesirable patterns and what triggers them. Develop a plan to change pessimism and negativity to optimistic hope. You can improve your habits, health, and live a more productive, meaningful life.

ESTABLISH HEALTHY HABITS

Most adults believe they are unchangeable. Have you ever said or heard someone else say, "That's just the way I am." But God created our minds with the ability to renew thoughts and change habits. Dr. Caroline Leaf believes it takes sixty-three days to form a new habit, not the twenty-one we've all heard of before.[2] Changing how you think takes time, so give yourself permission to start a journey knowing changes may take a while to become established. On a daily basis, evaluate every thought and dispel the defeating ones.

Creating new healthy habits begins in the mind. Our beliefs influence our decisions. If we understand why we believe eating unhealthy food is okay, we can alter our opinions and create a positive and healthy belief system. Part of this process is paying attention to what you put into your mind, not just your body.

Poor eating habits and lack of exercise are difficult behaviors to modify. To change a habit, you should gain the knowledge needed to alter your subconscious mind—your beliefs. Educate yourself on the reasons it is beneficial to eat healthy foods versus processed junk foods. Through learning which foods are healthy and which are not, you can promote positive eating habits.

Don't listen to food commercials or social media ads because they are trying to sell you more of their products. They don't care about your health. We can reverse years of propaganda about delicious fast food and junk food. Learn what is healthy so you can transform your belief system about food.

Many people cannot change their eating habits because they don't realize how the way they eat was ingrained in them for decades. Your family of origin may have eaten in an unhealthy manner, then passed those habits down to you. Know that you can change your diet and lifestyle. Pay attention to your thoughts and attitudes because they influence your choices.

Whatever beliefs you focus on, you will act upon. Reading the information in this book will help you choose to eat more of God's foods. As you do, your body receives the vitamins and minerals God designed to heal cells, which makes you look and feel younger.

Inputting positive lifestyle knowledge in your brain will change your mentality. As you learn, positive eating habits will naturally emerge. If you want to create a habit, do it consistently for over two months so it becomes part of your routine.

Another great way to gain knowledge, especially while you are working on changing your habits, is listening to healthy-living podcasts. If you type my name, Susan Neal, into a podcast app, loads of interviews will populate. Repeated exposure to positive content about healthy choices will cause this additional information to become a part of your new belief system. You will have the mental tools to implement this improved lifestyle successfully. You can change your future by changing the way you view the foods you eat.

When forming a new habit, the best thing to do is start small until you achieve success, then build from there. Begin with a written plan for implementing healthy habits. This strategy is in addition to your plan to resolve your root issue for being stuck. Planning brings mental clarity and peace. Determine what exercise works for you. Write down your healthy food choices and how you will prepare for healthy meals based on God's foods. When you don't have a plan, you feel less motivated.

Figure out where you are now and decide where you want to be. Create a vision of your goals and what you want your health, body, and life to look like. Do you want to lose a few pounds, increase your mobility, or gain muscle strength? Develop the steps to move forward, little by little. Set aside the next two months to change your unhealthy habits into positive ones.

The following tips will help you improve your health and well-being as you plan and work to achieve and maintain healthy living choices:

1. Write your attainable, measurable goals. Don't make the goal too big. Write the steps to achieve each goal. View your objective daily and focus on it.
2. Ask God to help you achieve your goals. Turn to the Lord for help when you struggle.
3. Place a Bible verse somewhere in your home to look at and recite when you need strength. I use Ephesians 5:18: "Don't drink too much wine, for many evils lie along that path; be filled instead with the Holy Spirit and controlled by him" (TLB). You can replace wine with any other unhealthy food, beverage, or habit.
4. Schedule your goal's steps into your life daily. For example, I schedule when I plan to walk or swim. At first, making changes is difficult, but after a while, they become routine, and you look forward to these new healthier habits.
5. Plan ahead for triggers and cravings that will prompt unwanted choices. Have healthy food on hand so you don't grab a bag of processed food.
6. Whenever you have a negative thought about yourself, replace it with a positive one.
7. At the end of each day, measure how you progressed in meeting your goal. For me, it's how many miles I walked or how long

I swam or if I worked out. Rate yourself with a self-measuring system such as one to five. Yesterday, I walked three miles, so I would give myself a five. If you don't measure it, you can't manage it.
8. Celebrate your achievements along the way and thank God for his help.
9. Share your goals with friends. When you do, momentum can come from your peers and social environment.
10. Find an accountability partner—a coach, friend, or trainer. Review how you're doing with them every week for an evaluation.
11. Get a buddy and go to the gym with them. This increases the likelihood that you'll go. Ask your partner to work with you on improving your eating habits. Partnership enhances motivation.
12. At the end of each week, evaluate what you did well and what you could improve. Develop a plan for the next week that includes your goals and routines.

Changing your habits requires repetition and recalibration. Practice your plan until it becomes second nature. When you eat poorly or don't work out, it is time to recalibrate—adjust your plan. Get back on track. During this time, ask God to strengthen you. Know that he loves you, and you are worthy of an abundant life. The new you will follow through with your plans and have self-respect.

After two months, these routines become habits you can continue for the rest of your life. This lifestyle change will help you age gracefully and live your life to the fullest.

SUMMARY

To some extent we are in control of our well-being through our daily healthy-living choices. Essential keys include renewing your mindset, healing emotionally, and resolving the root problem that contributes to harmful habits. Romans 12:2 says we can transform our minds: "Don't copy the behavior and customs of this world, but let God transform you into a new person by changing the way you think."

Recently, I visited the re-creation of Noah's Ark. It surprised me to find so many people in motorized wheelchairs. Now, many people have no choice due to things like injury, neurological issues, or birth defects, but I couldn't help wondering how many could have been spared that lot in life if they had access to the right food and exercise. We don't have to lose all of our body's physical abilities as we age.

We take our bodies for granted and fill them with all sorts of bad stuff. Over a lifetime, there is a cumulative effect. Chronic diseases caused by negative habits happen over a period of time. When we recognize that these behaviors are detrimental to our bodies, we can make changes before it's too late. We can do much to preserve our bodies and minds and look forward to healthier, longer lives.

Daily choices lead to either a healthy life or chronic illness. Do your negative lifestyle choices outnumber your positive ones? Choose to take control of your health—mind, body, and spirit. Live in alignment with the aspirational person you want to be, so you become that person God created you to be. With the help of Christ, you can!

Decide to make this the year you will be the healthiest you've ever been in your life. Raise your aspiration and vision, even if your health has been a challenge in the past. Take personal responsibility for your overall well-being. Accept the challenge. Demand more from yourself than you feel you have. Know that God created your body to work in a healthy way, and he will be with you in this journey. As you continue these new habits for the rest of your life, you will feel and look younger next year than you do today.

PERSONAL AND PRACTICAL APPLICATION

1. Do you feel you can't dig out of your unhealthy situation? In what way are you stuck?
2. Is the way you are living not serving you well? Do you have a root problem that is holding you back?

3. Do you have unhealed wounds from past trauma? Do you need to forgive someone?
4. Should you seek counseling? Who can you call to get help?
5. What negative habits do you turn to when you are anxious, stressed, or angry? What triggers your negative response?
6. Try to remember when each unwanted behavior began in your life and why. Was it in childhood, after a traumatic event, or after you believed a lie someone told you about yourself? Determine what caused the behavior.
7. What triggers your negative response? Keep track of these triggers in a journal or list.
8. List some alternate behaviors you could employ instead of your undesirable ones.
9. Brainstorm how you can prevent your negative response.
10. Evaluate your answers above and create a plan to change.

APPENDIX
FALL PREVENTION

Falls are the leading cause of injury and injury-related death in older adults aged sixty-five years and older. "One out of four older adults will fall each year in the United States." And of those falls, 20 percent cause an injury. Falls cause more than 95 percent of hip fractures, and most people who fall are women.[1]

Falls are not a normal part of aging, but all of us seem to fall occasionally in our life. The following precautions will help prevent falls:[2]

- Perform strength training exercises that strengthen your legs.
- Do exercises that improve balance, such as yoga, dance, or tai chi.
- Remove trip hazards, such a rugs, electrical cords, newspapers, boxes.
- Wear well-fitting shoes inside and outside the home.
- Store commonly used items on lower shelves.
- Use nonslip mats in the bathtub or shower.
- Add grab bars in the tub and next to the toilet.
- Purchase a shower seat to use when showering.
- Review medications you take that may cause dizziness or sleepiness.
- Get annual eye examinations and ensure your prescription glasses are up-to-date.
- Install handrails and lights on staircases.
- Improve the lighting in your home; install higher-wattage light bulbs.

- Install night-lights as needed.
- Make a clear path to light switches that are not near room entrances; install illuminated switches as needed.
- Do not climb ladders to replace light bulbs or retrieve an item (ask family or friends to help or hire someone).
- Store flashlights in an easily accessible place in case of a power outage.

Sensible footwear should be part of your fall-prevention plan. Don't wear flip-flops, floppy slippers, or high heels. Instead, wear well-fitted, flat, sturdy shoes with nonskid soles. Check out the soles of your shoes. If the soles have worn down to a flat surface, they are a tripping hazard. The cost of a pair of shoes is a lot less expensive than a hospital visit.

Many of these solutions are inexpensive and easy to implement. An investment in fall prevention will help you live independently longer. You can find the brochure "Check for Safety: A Home Fall Prevention Checklist for Older Adults" at https://www.cdc.gov/steadi/pdf/STEADI-Brochure-CheckForSafety-508.pdf.

NOTES

Introduction

1. Caroline Leaf, *Think and Eat Yourself Smart: A Neuroscientific Approach to a Sharper Mind and Healthier Life* (Ada, MI: Baker, 2016), 101–2.

1. Eat to Live Longer

1. Clara R. Freeman et al., "Impact of Sugar on the Body, Brain, and Behavior," *Frontiers in Bioscience (Landmark Edition)* 23, no. 12 (June 1, 2018): 2255–66, https://doi.org/10.2741/4704. PMID: 29772560.
2. Environmental Working Group, "Dirty Dozen," EWG's 2023 Shopper's Guide to Pesticides in Produce, 2023, https://www.ewg.org/foodnews/dirty-dozen.php.
3. Environmental Working Group, "Clean Fifteen," EWG's 2023 Shopper's Guide to Pesticides in Produce, 2023, https://www.ewg.org/foodnews/clean-fifteen.php.
4. Environmental Working Group, "Roundup for Breakfast, Part 2: In New Tests, Weed Killer Found in All Kids' Cereals Sampled," EWG.org, accessed October 4, 2023, https://www.ewg.org/news-insights/news-release/2018/10/roundup-breakfast-part-2-new-tests-weed-killer-found-all-kids.
5. Graham Brookes and Peter Barfoot, "Environmental Impacts of Genetically Modified (GM) Crop Use 1996–2016: Impacts on Pesticide Use and Carbon Emissions," *GM Crops & Food* 9, no. 3 (2018): 109–39, https://doi.org/10.1080/21645698.2018.1476792.
6. Brookes and Barfoot, "Environmental Impacts of GM Crop Use."
7. Holly Yan, "Jurors Give $289 Million to a Man They Say Got Cancer from Monsanto's Roundup Weedkiller," CNN Health, August 11, 2018, https://www.cnn.com/2018/08/10/health/monsanto-johnson-trial-verdict/index.html.
8. Centers for Disease Control and Prevention, "Leading Causes of Death," CDC.gov, https://www.cdc.gov/nchs/fastats/leading-causes-of-death.htm.
9. Julia Baudry et al, "Association of Frequency of Organic Food Consumption With Cancer Risk," *JAMA Internal Medicine* 178, no. 12 (2018), 1597.

10. National Pesticide Information Center, "Pesticide Ingredients Used in Organic Agriculture," NPIC.orst.edu, http://npic.orst.edu/ingred/organic.html; Ruby Tiwari and Ramdas Kanissery, "Organic Herbicide Options," Specialty Crop Grower, https://specialtycropgrower.com/florida-organic-herbicide-weeds/.
11. Bennett G. Childs et al., "Senescent Cells: An Emerging Target for Diseases of Ageing," *Nature Reviews. Drug Discovery* 16, no. 10 (2017): 718–35, https://doi.org/10.1038/nrd.2017.116.
12. Childs et al., "Senescent Cells."
13. Mohammad Bagherniya et al., "The Effect of Fasting or Calorie Restriction on Autophagy Induction: A Review of the Literature," *Ageing Research Reviews* 47 (2018): 183–97, https://doi.org/10.1016/j.arr.2018.08.004.
14. Cleveland Clinic, "Autophagy," https://my.clevelandclinic.org/health/articles/24058-autophagy.
15. Bagherniya et al., "Effect of Fasting."
16. Megan Forliti, "Mayo Researchers Extend Lifespan in Mice by As Much As 35 Percent," Mayo Clinic News Network, February 3, 2016, https://newsnetwork.mayoclinic.org/discussion/mayo-clinic-researchers-extend-lifespan-by-as-much-as-35-percent-in-mice-.
17. Forliti, "Mayo Researchers."
18. American Heart Association, "Added Sugars," https://www.heart.org/en/healthy-living/healthy-eating/eat-smart/sugar/added-sugars.
19. US Department of Agriculture, "Why Does the MyPlate.gov Website Include Tomatoes and Avocados in the Vegetable Group Instead of the Fruit Group?", USDA.gov, August 23, 2023, https://ask.usda.gov/s/article/Why-does-the-ChooseMyPlate-gov-website-include-tomatoes-and-avocados-in-the-Vegetable-Group-instead#:~:text=For%20example%2C%20tomatoes%2C%20avocados%2C,be%20vegetables%20rather%20than%20fruits.
20. Grain Foods Foundation, "The Milling Process," https://grainfoodsfoundation.org/grain-facts/the-milling-process/.
21. Centers for Disease Control ad Prevention, "About Chronic Diseases," https://www.cdc.gov/chronicdisease/index.htm.
22. Dorota Piasecka-Kwiatkowska et al., "Digestive Enzyme Inhibitors from Grains as Potential Components of Nutraceuticals," *Journal of Nutritional Science and Vitaminology* 58, no. 3 (2012): 217–20, https://doi.org/10.3177/jnsv.58.217.
23. Corey Whelan, "Brown Rice vs. White Rice: Which Is Better for You?", Healthline, September 29, 2018, https://www.healthline.com/health/food-nutrition/brown-rice-vs-white-rice.
24. Nicole M. Avena, Pedro Rada, and Bartley G. Hoebel, "Evidence for Sugar Addiction: Behavioral and Neurochemical Effects of Intermittent, Excessive

Sugar Intake," *Neuroscience and Biobehavioral Reviews* 32, no. 1 (2008): 20–39, https://doi.org/10.1016/j.neubiorev.2007.04.019; Leo Pruimboom, and Karin de Punder, "The Opioid Effects of Gluten Exorphins: Asymptomatic Celiac Disease," *Journal of Health, Population, and Nutrition* 33, no. 24 (November 24, 2015), https://doi.org/10.1186/s41043-015-0032-y.

25. "What Happens to Your Brain on Sugar, Explained by Science," MIC, last modified April 21, 2014, https://www.mic.com/articles/88015/what-happens-to-your-brain-on-sugar-explained-by-science.
26. Parul Dube, "Sweeteners and Their Glycemic Index: A Comparison," Healthifyme.com, October 14, 2022, https://www.healthifyme.com/blog/sweeteners-and-their-glycemic-index/.
27. Environmental Working Group, "Herbicides and GMO Crops," https://www.ewg.org/herbicides-and-gmo-crops.
28. Samvida Patel, "Which Sweeteners Rank Best and Worst on the Glycemic Index?", God Rx Health, July 19, 2023, https://www.goodrx.com/well-being/diet-nutrition/sweeteners; Glycemic Index, "High Fructose Corn Syrup vs. Sugar," https://www.glycemic-index.org/high-fructose-corn-syrup-vs-sugar.html.
29. John S. White, "Straight Talk About High-Fructose Corn Syrup: What It Is and What It Ain't," *The American Journal of Clinical Nutrition* 88, no. 6 (2008): 1716S–21S, https://doi.org/10.3945/ajcn.2008.25825B.
30. Alexandra Sifferlin, "Artificial Sweeteners Are Linked to Weight Gain—Not Weight Loss," *Time*, July 17, 2017, https://time.com/4859012/artificial-%20sweeteners-weight-loss/.
31. "Cancer: Carcinogenicity of the Consumption of Red Meat and Processed Meat," World Health Organization (WHO), accessed October 4, 2023, https://www.who.int/news-room/questions-and-answers/item/cancer-carcinogenicity-of-the-consumption-of-red-meat-and-processed-meat.
32. Eric Graber, "Are Omega-6 Polyunsaturated Fatty Acid-Rich Vegetable Oils Healthy?", American Society for Nutrition, September 24, 2020, https://nutrition.org/vegetable-oils/.
33. Ibrahim M. Dighriri et al., "Effects of Omega-3 Polyunsaturated Fatty Acids on Brain Functions: A Systematic Review," *Cureus* 14, no. 10 e30091 (October 9, 2022), https://doi.org/10.7759/cureus.30091.
34. Rachael Ajmera, "What Is Extra Virgin Olive Oil, and Why Is It Healthy?", Healthline, October 30, 2023, https://www.healthline.com/nutrition/extra-virgin-olive-oil.
35. Kris Gunnars, "Why Is Coconut Oil Good for You? A Healthy Oil for Cooking," Healthline, https://www.healthline.com/nutrition/why-is-coconut-oil-good-for-you.

Notes

36. US Food and Drug Administration, "Bisphenol A (BPA): Use in Food Contact Application," updated April 20, 2023, https://www.fda.gov/food/food-packaging-other-substances-come-contact-food-information-consumers/bisphenol-bpa-use-food-contact-application.
37. US Food and Drug Administration, "Bisphenol A (BPA)."
38. Roddy Scheer and Doug Moss, "Dirt Poor: Have Fruits and Vegetables Become Less Nutritious?", *Scientific American*, April 27, 2011, https://www.scientificamerican.com/article/soil-depletion-and-nutrition-loss/.
39. Katarzyna Maresz, "Proper Calcium Use: Vitamin K2 as a Promoter of Bone and Cardiovascular Health," *Integrative Medicine* (Encinitas, CA) 14, no. 1 (2015): 34–39, https://www.ncbi.nlm.nih.gov/pmc/articles/PMC4566462/.
40. Alshimaa M. El-Sheikh et al., "Relationship Between Trace Elements and Premature Graying," *International Journal of Trichology* 10, no. 6 (2018): 278, https://doi.org/10.4103/ijt.ijt_8_18. PMID: 30783336; PMCID: PMC6369637.
41. Cleveland Clinic, "Vitamin D Deficiency," https://my.clevelandclinic.org/health/diseases/15050-vitamin-d-vitamin-d-deficiency.
42. Fiona O'Leary and Samir Samman, "Vitamin B12 in Health and Disease," *Nutrients* 2, no. 3 (2010): 299–316, https://doi.org/10.3390/nu2030299.
43. National Heart, Lung, and Blood Institute, "Vitamin B12–Deficiency Anemia," updated March 24, 2022, https://www.nhlbi.nih.gov/health/anemia/vitamin-b12-deficiency-anemia.
44. Harvard T. H. Chan School of Public Health, "Magnesium," last reviewed March 2023, https://www.hsph.harvard.edu/nutritionsource/magnesium/#:~:text=RDA%3A%20The%20Recommended%20Dietary%20Allowance,cause%20harmful%20effects%20on%20health.
45. University of Nebraska—Lincoln, "8 Magnesium Deficiency Symptoms (and 9 High Magnesium Foods)," Nebraska Medicine University Health Center, https://health.unl.edu/8-magnesium-deficiency-symptoms-and-9-high-magnesium-foods.

2. Keep Your Gut Healthy

1. Hsin-Jung Wu and Eric Wu, "The Role of Gut Microbiota in Immune Homeostasis and Autoimmunity," *Gut Microbes* 3, no. 1 (2012): 4–14.
2. Wu and Wu, "Role of Gut Microbiota."
3. Cleveland Clinic, "How Your Gut Microbiome Impacts Your Health," June 8, 2022, https://health.clevelandclinic.org/gut-microbiome.
4. Cleveland Clinic, "How Your Gut Microbiome Impacts Your Health."

5. Mayo Clinic, "Helicobacter Pylori (H. pylori) Infection," May 5, 2022, https://www.mayoclinic.org/diseases-conditions/h-pylori/symptoms-causes/syc-20356171.
6. Mayo Clinic, "Helicobacter Pylori (H. pylori) Infection."
7. Hannah Kleinfeld, "Candida and Probiotics: Keeping Yeast Overgrowths in Check," Omnibiotic, https://www.omnibioticlife.com/candida-and-probiotics/.
8. Kleinfeld, "Candida and Probiotics."
9. Weill Cornell Medicine, "Toxin-Producing Yeast Strains in Gut Fuel IBD," Science Daily, March 16, 2022, www.sciencedaily.com/releases/2022/03/220316145804.htm.
10. Kleinfeld, "Candida and Probiotics."
11. Pushpanathan Muthuirulan, "Leaky Gut Syndrome: Mystery Illness Triggered by *Candida albicans*," *Journal of Nutritional Health & Food Engineering* 4, no. 3 (May 2016): 448–49, https://doi.org/10.15406/jnhfe.2016.04.00133.
12. Amy Myers, "Candida Overgrowth: 10 Signs and the Best Solution," Amy Myers MD, https://www.amymyersmd.com/article/signs-candida-overgrowth.
13. Myers, "Candida Overgrowth."
14. Myers, "Candida Overgrowth."
15. Neuroscience News, "Link Between Alzheimer's Disease and Gut Microbiota Is Confirmed," last modified November 13, 2020, https://neurosciencenews.com/microbiome-alzheimers-17273/.
16. Muthuirulan, "Leaky Gut Syndrome."
17. WebMD, "What Is Hypochlorhydria," WebMD.com, November 15, 2021, reviewed by Dan Brennan, MD, https://www.webmd.com/digestive-disorders/what-is-hypochlorhydria.
18. Alexander Rinehart, "The Domino Effect of Stomach Acid on Digestion and the Gut Microbiome," Dr. Alex Rinehart, July 29, 2020, https://dralexrinehart.com/articles/the-domino-effect-of-stomach-acid-on-digestion-and-the-gut-microbiome/.
19. Najate Achamrah, Perrie Déchelotte, and Moïse Coëffier, "Glutamine and the Regulation of Intestinal Permeability: From Bench to Bedside," Current Opinion in Clinical Nutrition and Metabolic Care 20, no. 1 (2017): 86–91, https://doi.org/10.1097/MCO.0000000000000339.
20. Centers for Disease Control and Prevention, "Adult Obesity Facts," last reviewed, May 17, 2022, https://www.cdc.gov/obesity/data/adult.html; Centers for Disease Control and Prevention, "Chronic Diseases in America," last reviewed December 13, 2022, https://www.cdc.gov/chronicdisease/resources/infographic/chronic-diseases.htm.
21. P. Rada, N. M. Avena, and B. G. Hoebel, "Daily Bingeing on Sugar Repeatedly Releases Dopamine in the Accumbens Shell," *Neuroscience* 134, no. 3 (2005): 737–44, https://doi.org/10.1016/j.neuroscience.2005.04.043.

22. The Facebook page can be found at https://www.facebook.com/groups/184355458927013. My book is found anywhere books are sold. Susan U. Neal, *7 Steps to Get Off Sugar and Carbohydrates* (Pensacola: Christian Indie Publishing, 2017).
23. Jing Kang, Austin Scholp, and Jack J. Jiang, "A Review of the Physiological Effects and Mechanisms of Singing," *Journal of Voice : Official Journal of the Voice Foundation* 32, no. 4 (2018): 390–95, https://doi.org/10.1016/j.jvoice.2017.07.008.
24. Davis Cammann et al, "Genetic correlations between Alzheimer's disease and gut microbiome genera," *Scientific Reports* 13, no. 1 (2023).
25. American Heart Association, "How Much Sugar Is Too Much?", https://www.heart.org/en/healthy-living/healthy-eating/eat-smart/sugar/how-much-sugar-is-too-much.
26. Izzah Vasim, Chaudry N. Majeed, and Mark D. DeBoer, "Intermittent Fasting and Metabolic Health," *Nutrients* 14, no. 3 (January 31, 2022): 631, https://doi.org/10.3390/nu14030631.
27. Aaron Kandola and Mandy French, "What Are the Benefits of Intermittent Fasting?", Medical News Today, November 29, 2023, https://www.medicalnewstoday.com/articles/323605.
28. Vasim et al., "Intermittent Fasting and Metabolic Health"; University of Illinois at Chicago, "Research Review Shows Intermittent Fasting Works for Weight Loss, Health Changes," ScienceDaily, accessed January 29, 2024, www.sciencedaily.com/releases/2021/10/211012102652.htm.
29. University of Illinois at Chicago, "Research Review Shows Intermittent Fasting Works for Weight Loss, Health Changes."
30. Kris Gunnars, "What Is Intermittent Fasting and How Does It Work?", Healthline, October 31, 2023, https://www.healthline.com/nutrition/10-health-benefits-of-intermittent-fasting.
31. Kandola and French, "What Are the Benefits of Intermittent Fasting?"
32. Vasim et al., "Intermittent Fasting and Metabolic Health."
33. Sophie C. Killer, Andrew K. Blannin, and Asker E. Jeukendrup, "No Evidence of Dehydration with Moderate Daily Coffee Intake: A Counterbalanced Cross-Over Study in a Free-Living Population," *PLOS One* 9, no. 1 e84154 (January 9, 2014), https://doi.org/10.1371/journal.pone.0084154.
34. Myers, "Candida Overgrowth."

3. The Secret to Staying Physically Active

1. Dr. Peter J. D'Adamo, *Eat Right 4 Your Type: The Individualized Blood Type Diet Solution* (New York: Berkley, 1996).

2. National Center for Complementary and Integrative Health, "Yoga: What You Need to Know," National Institutes of Health, August 2023, https://www.nccih.nih.gov/health/yoga-what-you-need-to-know.
3. C. M. Snow et al., "Long-Term Exercise Using Weighted Vests Prevents Hip Bone Loss in Postmenopausal Women," *The Journals of Gerontology. Series A, Biological Sciences and Medical Sciences* 55, no. 9 (2000): M489–91, https://doi.org/10.1093/gerona/55.9.m489.
4. College of Naturopathic Medicine, "Rebounding: Miracle Exercise that Transforms Health," https://www.naturopathy-uk.com/news/blog/2023/04/19/rebounding-miracle-exercise-that-transforms-health/#:~:text=Rebounding%20can%20provide%20a%20great,nutrients%20to%20reach%20your%20cells.
5. Mayo Clinic, "Strength Training: Get Stronger, Leaner, Healthier," April 29, 2023, https://www.mayoclinic.org/healthy-lifestyle/fitness/in-depth/strength-training/art-20046670.
6. Mayo Clinic, "Strength Training."
7. Mayo Clinic, "Strength Training."
8. Permanente Medicine, "Regular Exercise Benefits Both Mind and Body: A Psychiatrist Explains," Mid-Atlantic Permanente Medical Group, December 22, 2021, https://mydoctor.kaiserpermanente.org/mas/news/regular-exercise-benefits-both-mind-and-body-a-psychiatrist-explains-1903986.
9. Cleveland Clinic, "Shoes Getting Tight? Why Your Feet Change Size Over Time," September 18, 2022, https://health.clevelandclinic.org/shoes-getting-tight-feet-change-size-time.

4. Keep Your Brain Young

1. Centers for Disease Control and Prevention, "About Dementia," April 5, 2019, https://www.cdc.gov/aging/dementia/index.html.
2. Centers for Disease Control and Prevention, "About Dementia."
3. Shazia Jatoi et al., "Low Vitamin B12 Levels: An Underestimated Cause of Minimal Cognitive Impairment and Dementia," *Cureus* 12, no. 2 (February 13, 2012): e6976, https://doi.org/10.7759/cureus.6976.
4. Mayo Clinic, "Vascular Dementia," July 29, 2021, https://www.mayoclinic.org/diseases-conditions/vascular-dementia/symptoms-causes/syc-20378793.
5. Alzheimer's Association, "2019 Alzheimer's Disease Facts and Figures Report," accessed October 4, 2023, pages 17, 25, https://www.alz.org/media/Documents/alzheimers-facts-and-figures-2019-r.pdf.
6. National Institute on Aging, "What Causes Alzheimer's Disease?", National Institutes of Health, December 24, 2019, https://www.nia.nih.gov/health/alzheimers-causes-and-risk-factors/what-causes-alzheimers-disease.

Notes

7. Dale Bredesen, *The End of Alzheimer's Program: The First Protocol to Enhance Cognition and Reverse Decline at Any Age* (New York: Avery, 2022), 16–17.
8. Bredesen, *End of Alzheimer's Program.*
9. Thomas Campbell, "A Plant-Based Diet and Stroke," *Journal of Geriatric Cardiology* 14, no. 5 (May 2017): 321–26, https://doi.org/10.11909/j.issn.1671-5411.2017.05.010.
10. Jean A. Welsh et al., "Production-Related Contaminants (Pesticides, Antibiotics and Hormones) in Organic and Conventionally Produced Milk Samples Sold in the USA," *Public Health Nutrition* 22, no. 16 (2019): 2972–80, https://doi.org/10.1017/S136898001900106X.
11. Christopher Masterjohn, "Fatty Acid Analysis of Grass-Fed and Grain-Fed Beef Tallow," The Weston A. Price Foundation, January 21, 2014, https://www.westonaprice.org/health-topics/know-your-fats/fatty-acid-analysis-of-grass-fed-and-grain-fed-beef-tallow/#gsc.tab=0.
12. Austin Perlmutter, "Why Fat Matters for Your Brain Health," Austin Perlmutter MD, May 29, 2023, https://www.austinperlmutter.com/post/why-fat-matters-for-your-brain-health; Campbell, "A Plant-Based Diet and Stroke."
13. Charles Schmidt, "Inflammation and Brain Health," Harvard Medicine, Autumn 2021, https://magazine.hms.harvard.edu/articles/inflammation-and-brain-health.
14. Roma Pahwa, Amandeep Goyal, and Ishwarlal Jialal, "Chronic Inflammation," National Institutes of Health, August 7, 2023, https://www.ncbi.nlm.nih.gov/books/NBK493173/.
15. Jefferson W. Kinney et al., "Inflammation as a Central Mechanism in Alzheimer's Disease," *Alzheimer's & Dementia (New York, NY)* 4 (September 6, 2018): 575–90, https://doi.org/10.1016/j.trci.2018.06.014.
16. Brenna Cholerton et al., "Type 2 Diabetes, Cognition, and Dementia in Older Adults: Toward a Precision Health Approach," *Diabetes Spectrum: a Publication of the American Diabetes Association* 29, no. 4 (2016): 210–19, https://doi.org/10.2337/ds16-0041.
17. Thuy Trang Nguyen et al., "Type 3 Diabetes and Its Role Implications in Alzheimer's Disease," *International Journal of Molecular Sciences* 21, no. 9 (April 30, 2020): 3165, https://doi.org/10.3390/ijms21093165.
18. Thomas Ball, "The Top 10 Inflammatory Foods to Avoid," Performance Health Center, February 4, 2020, https://performancehealthcenter.com/2020/02/the-top-10-inflammatory-foods-to-avoid/.
19. Bredesen, *End of Alzheimer's Program*, 93–95.
20. Mohammad Bagheriniya et al., "The Effect of Fasting or Calorie Restriction on Autophagy Induction: Review of the Literature," *Ageing Research Reviews* 47 (November 2018): 183–97, https://www.sciencedirect.com/science/article/abs/pii/S1568163718301478?via%3Dihub.

21. Bredesen, *End of Alzheimer's Program*, 20.
22. Bredesen, *End of Alzheimer's Program*, 20.
23. Rena Kyriakides, Patrick Jones, and Bhaskar K. Somani, "Role of D-Mannose in the Prevention of Recurrent Urinary Tract Infections: Evidence from a Systematic Review of the Literature," *European Urology Focus* 7, no. 5 (September 21, 2021): 1166–69, https://doi.org/10.1016/j.euf.2020.09.004.
24. Bredesen, *End of Alzheimer's Program*, 25.
25. Kelsey Kidd, "6 Tips to Keep Your Brain Healthy," Mayo Clinic Health System, December 29, 2022, https://www.mayoclinichealthsystem.org/hometown-health/speaking-of-health/5-tips-to-keep-your-brain-healthy.
26. "Exercise and Your Arteries," *Harvard Health*, July 31, 2023, https://www.health.harvard.edu/heart-health/exercise-and-your-arteries.
27. Centers for Disease Control and Prevention, "Physical Activity Boosts Brain Health," last reviewed: February 24, 2023, https://www.cdc.gov/nccdphp/dnpao/features/physical-activity-brain-health/index.html.
28. Prerna Sangle et al., "Vitamin B12 Supplementation: Preventing Onset and Improving Prognosis of Depression," *Cureus* 12, no. 10 (October 26, 2020): e11169, https://doi.org/10.7759/cureus.11169.
29. Ali Niklewicz et al., "The Importance of Vitamin B12 for Individuals Choosing Plant-Based Diets," *European Journal of Nutrition* 62, no. 3 (2023): 1551–59, https://doi.org/10.1007/s00394-022-03025-4.
30. Donald R. Davis, "Declining Fruit and Vegetable Nutrient Composition: What Is the Evidence?", *HortScience horts* 44, no. 1 (2009): 15–19, https://doi.org/10.21273/HORTSCI.44.1.15.
31. Patrice Sutton et al., "Toxic Environmental Chemicals: The Role of Reproductive Health Professionals in Preventing Harmful Exposures," *American Journal of Obstetrics and Gynecology* 207, no. 3 (2012): 164–73, https://doi.org/10.1016/j.ajog.2012.01.034.
32. Manivannan Yegambaram et al., "Role of Environmental Contaminants in the Etiology of Alzheimer's Disease: A Review," *Current Alzheimer Research* 12, no. 2 (2015): 116–46, https://doi.org/10.2174/1567205012666150204121719.
33. Rebecca Robbins et al., "Examining Sleep Deficiency and Disturbance and Their Risk for Incident Dementia and All-Cause Mortality in Older Adults Across 5 Years in the United States," *Aging* 13 (February 11, 2021): 3254–68, https://doi.org/10.18632/aging.202591.
34. Myuri Ruthirakuhan et al., "Use of Physical and Intellectual Activities and Socialization in the Management of Cognitive Decline of Aging and in Dementia: A Review," *Journal of Aging Research* 2012 (2012): 384875, https://doi.org/10.1155/2012/384875.
35. Bredesen, *End of Alzheimer's Program*, 35–47, 200, 239–48.

Notes

36. Bredesen, *End of Alzheimer's Program*, 31.
37. Rammohan V. Rao et al., "Rationale for a Multi-Factorial Approach for the Reversal of Cognitive Decline in Alzheimer's Disease and MCI: A Review," *International Journal of Molecular Sciences* 24, no. 2 (January 14, 2023): 1659, https://doi.org/10.3390/ijms24021659.
38. Mather Hospital, "The Connection Between Heart Health & Dementia," https://www.matherhospital.org/wellness-at-mather/the-connection-between-heart-health-dementia/.

5. Eliminate Toxins: Inside and Out

1. Patrice Sutton et al., "Toxic Environmental Chemicals: The Role of Reproductive Health Professionals in Preventing Harmful Exposures," *American Journal of Obstetrics and Gynecology* 207, no. 3 (2012): 164–73, https://doi.org/10.1016/j.ajog.2012.01.034.
2. Aolin Wang et al., "Suspect Screening, Prioritization, and Confirmation of Environmental Chemicals in Maternal-Newborn Pairs from San Francisco," *Environmental Science & Technology* 55, no. 8 (2021): 5037–49.
3. Lillian Zhou and Julia Martiner, "Personal Care Product Chemicals Banned in Europe but Still Found in U.S.," Environmental Working Group, October 25, 2022, https://www.ewg.org/news-insights/news/2022/10/personal-care-product-chemicals-banned-europe-still-found-us#:~:text=The%20EU%20and%20other%20countries,banned%2024%20chemicals%20from%20cosmetics.
4. Susan Cosier, "Mercury's Journey from Coal-Burning Power Plants to Your Plate," National Resources Defense Council, May 2, 2023, https://www.nrdc.org/stories/mercurys-journey-coal-burning-power-plants-your-plate.
5. Dale Bredesen, *The End of Alzheimer's Program: The First Protocol to Enhance Cognition and Reverse Decline at Any Age* (New York: Avery, 2022), 271.
6. Ashley J. Malin, "Fluoride Exposure and Thyroid Function Among Adults Living in Canada: Effect Modification by Iodine Status," *Environment International* 121, no. 1 (December 2018): 667–74; Aishwarya Nathan, "Effect of Chlorine Water Consumption on Phenotypic and Microbiome Development," Rutgers University Libraries (2019), https://doi.org/10.7282/t3-a9s4-kp69.
7. Keiken Engineering, "Reverse Osmosis vs. Carbon Filter: How Does It Work?," April 2023, https://www.keiken-engineering.com/news/reverse-osmosis-vs-carbon-filter-how-does-it-work.
8. Sandee LaMotte, "Bottled Water Contains Thousands of Nanoplastics So Small They Can Invade the Body's Cells, Study Says," CNN, January 8, 2024,

https://www.cnn.com/2024/01/08/health/bottled-water-nanoplastics-study-wellness/index.html.
9. Erin Jackson et al., "Adipose Tissue as a Site of Toxin Accumulation," *Comprehensive Physiology* 7, no. 4 (September 12, 2017): 1085–135, https://doi.org/10.1002/cphy.c160038.
10. Oana Mărgărita Ghimpețeanu et al., "Antibiotic Use in Livestock and Residues in Food-A Public Health Threat: A Review," *Foods (Basel, Switzerland)* 11, no. 10 (May 16, 2022): 1430, https://doi.org/10.3390/foods11101430; Steven Wright, "Antibiotics in Grain-Fed Meat: What You Need to Know," Healthy Gut, https://healthygut.com/antibiotics-in-grain-fed-meat/.
11. Theocharis Konstantinidis et al., "Effects of Antibiotics upon the Gut Microbiome: A Review of the Literature," *Biomedicines* 8, no. 11 (November 16, 2020): 502, https://doi.org/10.3390/biomedicines8110502.
12. Mohammed M. Qaid and Khalid A. Abdoun, "Safety and Concerns of Hormonal Application in Farm Animal Production: A Review," *Journal of Applied Animal Research* 50, no. 1 (June 24, 2022): 426–39, https://doi.org/10.1080/09712119.2022.2089149.
13. "Cancer: Carcinogenicity of the Consumption of Red Meat and Processed Meat," World Health Organization (WHO), accessed October 4, 2023, https://www.who.int/news-room/questions-and-answers/item/cancer-carcinogenicity-of-the-consumption-of-red-meat-and-processed-meat.
14. Katarzyna Madej, Tatyana K. Kalenik, and Wojciech Piekoszewski, "Sample Preparation and Determination of Pesticides in Fat-Containing Foods," *Food Chemistry* 269 (December 15, 2018): 527–41, https://www.sciencedirect.com/science/article/abs/pii/S0308814618311476?via%3Dihub.
15. Grazia Barone et al., "Levels of Mercury, Methylmercury and Selenium in Fish: Insights into Children Food Safety," *Toxics* 9, no. 2 (February 20, 2021): 39, https://doi.org/10.3390/toxics9020039.
16. US Food and Drug Administration, "Dental Amalgam Fillings," last updated February 18, 2021, https://www.fda.gov/medical-devices/dental-devices/dental-amalgam-fillings.
17. Institute for Systemic Dentistry, "Safe Mercury Amalgam Removal," https://holisticdentistrynj.com/safe-amalgam-mercury-removal/; Robin Warwick et al., "Mercury Vapour Exposure During Dental Student Training in Amalgam Removal," *Journal of Occupational Medicine and Toxicology (London, England)* 8, no. 1 (October 3, 2013): 27, https://doi.org/10.1186/1745-6673-8-27.
18. Centers for Disease Control and Prevention, "Lead in Paint," last reviewed December 16, 2022, https://www.cdc.gov/nceh/lead/prevention/sources/paint.htm.

Notes

19. John E. Schjenken et al., "Endocrine Disruptor Compounds—A Cause of Impaired Immune Tolerance Driving Inflammatory Disorders of Pregnancy?", *Frontiers in Endocrinology* 12 (2021).
20. Plaine Products, "Why We Need to Understand the History of Plastic Before We Can Tackle the Problem," https://www.plaineproducts.com/why-we-need-to-understand-the-history-of-plastic-before-we-can-tackle-the-problem/.
21. Minnesota Department of Health, "Bisphenol A," last updated January 25, 2023, https://www.health.state.mn.us/communities/environment/risk/chemhazard/bisphenola.html.
22. Tricorbraun, "What Does BPA-Free Mean and Is It Safe?", https://www.tricorbraun.com/blog/what-does-bpa-free-mean-and-is-it-safe.html.
23. Miriam J. Woodward et al., "Phthalates and Sex Steroid Hormones Among Men From NHANES, 2013–2016," *The Journal of Clinical Endocrinology & Metabolism* 105, no. 4 (2020): e1225–34.
24. Yvette Shen, Phthalate Regulations in the European Union: An Overview," Compliance Gate, May 15, 2023, https://www.compliancegate.com/phthalate-regulations-european-union/; Paulina Campos, "9 Beauty Ingredients that Are Banned in Europe (But Legal in the US)," Byrdie, January 28, 2022, https://www.byrdie.com/banned-ingredients-europe.
25. Lariah Edwards et al., "Phthalate and Novel Plasticizer Concentrations in Food Items from U.S. Fast Food Chains: A Preliminary Analysis," *Journal of Exposure Science & Environmental Epidemiology* 32 (2022): 366–73, https://doi.org/10.1038/s41370-021-00392-8.
26. Yunxiao Yang et al., "Detection of Various Microplastics in Patients Undergoing Cardiac Surgery," *Environmental Science & Technology* 57, no. 30 (July 13, 2023): 10911–18, https://doi.org/10.1021/acs.est.2c07179.
27. Judita Zymantiene et al., "Effect of electromagnetic field exposure on mouse brain morphological and histopathological profiling," *Journal of Veterinary Research* 64, no. 2 (2020): 319–24.
28. Vest Tech, "What You Don't Know About Wearable Tech Radiation Exposure," https://vesttech.com/what-you-dont-know-about-wearable-tech-radiation-exposure/.
29. Erica Cirino, "Should You Be Worried About EMF Exposure?", Healthline, December 8, 2023, https://www.healthline.com/health/emf.
30. Green Science Policy Institute "Consumer Resources," https://greensciencepolicy.org/resources/consumer-resources/.
31. Jacquelyn Cafasso, "Are Dryer Sheets Safe to Use?", Healthline, September 18, 2019, https://www.healthline.com/health/dryer-sheets-toxicity.
32. Monica Amarelo, Study: Replacing Furniture and Foam Reduces Levels of Toxic Flame Retardants," Environmental Working Group, March 24, 2021,

https://www.ewg.org/news-insights/news-release/2021/03/study-replacing-furniture-and-foam-reduces-levels-toxic-flame.
33. Jackson et al., "Adipose Tissue as a Site of Toxin Accumulation."
34. Shilpa S. Shetty et al., "Environmental Pollutants and Their Effects on Human Health," *Heliyon* 9, no. 9 (September 2023): e19496, https://doi.org/10.1016/j.heliyon.2023.e19496.
35. Sutton et al., "Toxic Environmental Chemicals."
36. Bonafide, "Top 10 Foods for Detoxification," January 9, 2020, https://www.bonafideprovisions.com/blogs/blog/top-10-foods-for-detoxification.
37. Mount Sinai, "Milk Thistle," https://www.mountsinai.org/health-library/herb/milk-thistle.
38. Manouchehr Khoshbaten et al., "N-Acetylcysteine Improves Liver Function in Patients with Non-Alcoholic Fatty Liver Disease," *Hepatitis Monthly* 10, no. 1 (2010): 12–16; Corey Whelan, "Glutathione Benefits," Healthline, April 18, 2023, https://www.healthline.com/health/glutathione-benefits.
39. Orlando M. Gutiérrez, "Sodium- and Phosphorus-Based Food Additives: Persistent but Surmountable Hurdles in the Management of Nutrition in Chronic Kidney Disease," *Advances in Chronic Kidney Disease* 20, no. 2 (2013): 150–56, https://doi.org/10.1053/j.ackd.2012.10.008.
40. Michelle Vallet, "Updates in Research: Manual Lymphatic Drainage," American Massage Therapy Association, May 1, 2023, https://www.amtamassage.org/publications/massage-therapy-journal/research-update-lymph-drainage/.
41. Asutra, "Magnesium Flakes vs. Epsom Salts," https://asutra.com/blogs/asutra-life/magnesium-flakes-vs-epson-salts.
42. Ronni Gordon, "The Benefits and Risks of Dry Brushing," Healthline, March 14, 2023, https://www.healthline.com/health/dry-brushing.
43. Ask the Scientists, "Your Detox Organs Need Dietary Fiber," https://askthescientists.com/qa/dietary-fiber-and-detox-organs/; Mayo Clinic, "Dietary Fiber: Essential for a Healthy Diet," November 4, 2022, https://www.mayoclinic.org/healthy-lifestyle/nutrition-and-healthy-eating/in-depth/fiber/art-20043983.
44. Wen-Hui Kuan, Yi-Lang Chen, and Chao-Lin Liu, "Excretion of Ni, Pb, Cu, As, and Hg in Sweat Under Two Sweating Conditions," *International Journal of Environmental Research and Public Health* 19, no. 7 (April 4, 2022): 4323, https://doi.org/10.3390/ijerph19074323.
45. Jonathan Vellinga, "Can Saunas Really Help You Become Healthier?", Temecula Center for Integrative Medicine, January 4, 2022, https://www.tcimedicine.com/post/can-saunas-really-help-you-become-healthier.

46. Joy Hussain and Marc Cohen, "Clinical Effects of Regular Dry Sauna Bathing: A Systematic Review," *Evidence-Based Complementary and Alternative Medicine: eCAM* (April 24, 2018), https://doi.org/10.1155/2018/1857413.
47. Margaret E. Sears, Kathleen J. Kerr, and Riina I. Bray, "Arsenic, Cadmium, Lead, and Mercury in Sweat: A Systematic Review," *Journal of Environmental and Public Health* (2012), https://doi.org/10.1155/2012/184745.
48. Jessica Griffiths, "Are Saunas Good for Your Skin? Here's What We Found Out," Dermstore, https://www.dermstore.com/blog/are-saunas-good-for-your-skin/; Pure Medical, "Infrared Sauna for Cellulite," https://pure-medical.co.uk/infra-red-sauna-therapy/infrared-sauna-for-cellulite.
49. Tanjaniina Laukkanen et al., "Association Between Sauna Bathing and Fatal Cardiovascular and All-Cause Mortality Events," *JAMA Internal Medicine* 175, no. 4 (April 2015): 542–48, https://doi.org/10.1001/jamainternmed.2014.8187.
50. Laukkanen et al., "Association Between Sauna Bathing and Fatal Cardiovascular . . . Events."
51. Pure Medical, "Infrared Sauna for Cellulite."
52. Laukkanen et al., "Association Between Sauna Bathing and Fatal Cardiovascular . . . Events."
53. Louisa Flintoft, "Identical Twins: Epigenetics Makes the Difference," *Nature Reviews Genetics* 6, no. 667 (August 10, 2005), https://doi.org/10.1038/nrg1693.
54. Jorge Alejandro Alegría-Torres, Andrea Baccarelli, and Valentina Bollati, "Epigenetics and Lifestyle," *Epigenomics* 3, no. 3 (2011): 267–77, https://doi.org/10.2217/epi.11.22.
55. National Human Genome Research Institute, "Epigenomics Fact Sheet," last updated August 16, 2020, https://www.genome.gov/about-genomics/fact-sheets/Epigenomics-Fact-Sheet.
56. Centers for Disease Control and Prevention, "What Is Epigenetics?", last updated August 15, 2022, https://www.cdc.gov/genomics/disease/epigenetics.htm.
57. Sara Velilla et al., "Smoking and Age-Related Macular Degeneration: Review and Update," *Journal of Ophthalmology* 2013 (2013): 895147, https://doi.org/10.1155/2013/895147.
58. "BRCA Gene Mutations: Cancer Risk and Genetic Testing," National Cancer Institute, accessed October 5, 2023, https://www.cancer.gov/about-cancer/causes-prevention/genetics/brca-fact-sheet.
59. Tommy Nyberg et al., "Prostate Cancer Risks for Male BRCA1 and BRCA2 Mutation Carriers: A Prospective Cohort Study," *European Urology* 77, no. 1 (2020): 24–35, https://doi.org/10.1016/j.eururo.2019.08.025.
60. Alegría-Torres, Baccarelli, and Bollati, "Epigenetics and Lifestyle."
61. Centers for Disease Control and Prevention, "What Is Epigenetics?"

6. Balance and Stabilize Your Hormones

1. Mauri José Piazza and Almir Antônio Urbanetz, "Environmental Toxins and the Impact of Other Endocrine Disrupting Chemicals in Women's Reproductive Health," *JBRA Assisted Reproduction* 23, no. 2 (April 30, 2019): 154–64, https://doi.org/10.5935/1518-0557.20190016; Alice Park, "Menopause Makes Your Body Age Faster," *Time*, July 25, 2016, https://time.com/4422860/menopause-accelerates-aging/.
2. Ariane Lang, "10 Natural Ways to Balance Your Hormones," Healthline, August 7, 2023, https://www.healthline.com/nutrition/balance-hormones.
3. Cleveland Clinic, "Hormones," last reviewed February 23, 2023, https://my.clevelandclinic.org/health/articles/22464-hormones.
4. Mayo Clinic, "Menopause," May 25, 2023, https://www.mayoclinic.org/diseases-conditions/menopause/symptoms-causes/syc-20353397.
5. Matthew Lee Smith et al., "Sexually Transmitted Infection Knowledge Among Older Adults: Psychometrics and Test-Retest Reliability," *International Journal of Environmental Research and Public Health* 17, no. 7 (April 3, 2020): 2462, https://doi.org/10.3390/ijerph17072462.
6. "Cervical Cancer Statistics," Centers for Disease Control and Prevention, last modified June 8, 2023, https://www.cdc.gov/cancer/cervical/statistics/index.htm.
7 "Cervical Cancer Statistics."
8. Tampa General Hospital, "Endocrine Disorders," https://www.tgh.org/institutes-and-services/conditions/endocrine-disorder.
9. Cleveland Clinic, "Perimenopause," last reviewed October 5, 2021, https://my.clevelandclinic.org/health/diseases/21608-perimenopause.
10. Bill L. Lasley, S. Crawford, and D. S. McConnell, "Adrenal Androgens and the Menopausal Transition," *Obstetrics and Gynecology Clinics of North America* 38, no. 3 (2011): 467–75, https://doi.org/10.1016/j.ogc.2011.06.001; James L. Wilson, *Adrenal Fatigue: The 21st Century Stress Syndrome* (Petaluma, CA: Smart Publications, 2001), 17–19.
11. Cleveland Clinic, "Menopause," last reviewed October 5, 2021, https://my.clevelandclinic.org/health/diseases/21841-menopause.
12. Salama Alblooshi et al., "Does Menopause Elevate the Risk for Developing Depression and Anxiety? Results from a Systematic Review," *Australasian Psychiatry: Bulletin of Royal Australian and New Zealand College of Psychiatrists* 31, no. 2 (2023): 165–73, https://doi.org/10.1177/10398562231165439.
13. Sara Beth Cichowski, "UTIs After Menopause: Why They're Common and What to Do About Them," American College of Obstetricians and Gynecologists, last reviewed November 2023, https://www.acog.org/womens-health/experts-and-stories/the-latest/utis-after-menopause-why-theyre-common-and-what-to-do-about-them.

Notes

14. Mayo Clinic, "Osteoporosis," September 7, 2023, https://www.mayoclinic.org/diseases-conditions/osteoporosis/symptoms-causes/syc-20351968.
15. NHS Inform, "Bone Health and Falls," last updated March 14, 2023, https://www.nhsinform.scot/healthy-living/preventing-falls/keeping-well/bone-health-and-falls/.
16. Mayo Clinic, "Osteoporosis."
17. Harvard Health Publishing, "Strength Training Builds More than Muscles," Harvard Medical School, January 16, 2024, https://www.health.harvard.edu/staying-healthy/strength-training-builds-more-than-muscles.
18. Mark Goepel et al., "Urinary Incontinence in the Elderly: Part 3 of a Series of Articles on Incontinence," *Deutsches Arzteblatt International* 107, no. 30 (2010): 531–36, https://doi.org/10.3238/arztebl.2010.0531.
19. Mayo Clinic, "Kegel Exercises: A How-to Guide for Women," December 6, 2022, https://www.mayoclinic.org/healthy-lifestyle/womens-health/in-depth/kegel-exercises/art-20045283.
20. Mayo Clinic, "Male Menopause: Myth or Reality?", May 24, 2022, https://www.mayoclinic.org/healthy-lifestyle/mens-health/in-depth/male-menopause/art-20048056; Cleveland Clinic, "Low Testosterone (Male Hypogonadism)," last reviewed September 2, 2022, https://my.clevelandclinic.org/health/diseases/15603-low-testosterone-male-hypogonadism.
21. Biagio Barone et al., "The Role of Testosterone in the Elderly: What Do We Know?", *International Journal of Molecular Sciences* 23, no. 7 (2022): 3535.
22. Cleveland Clinic, "Low Testosterone (Male Hypogonadism)."
23. Andriy Yabluchanskiy and Panayiotis D. Tsitouras, "Is Testosterone Replacement Therapy in Older Men Effective and Safe?", *Drugs & Aging* 36, no. 11 (2019): 981–89.
24. "Low Testosterone (Male Hypogonadism)," Cleveland Clinic, accessed October 5, 2023, https://my.clevelandclinic.org/health/diseases/15603-low-testosterone-male-hypogonadism.
25. Kathryn Whitbourne, "Adrenal Fatigue: Is It Real?", WebMD, last reviewed September 18, 2023, https://www.webmd.com/a-to-z-guides/adrenal-fatigue-is-it-real.
26. Bill L. Lasley, S. Crawford, and D. S. McConnell, "Adrenal Androgens and the Menopausal Transition," *Obstetrics and Gynecology Clinics of North America* 38, no. 3 (2011): 467–75, https://doi.org/10.1016/j.ogc.2011.06.001.
27. Women's Health Network, "What Is Adrenal Fatigue? Symptoms, Causes, and Natural Treatment for Women," reviewed by Dr. Sharon Stills, NMD, https://www.womenshealthnetwork.com/adrenal-fatigue-and-stress/.
28. Anju Mathur, "How Modern Lifestyles Are Leading to Adrenal Fatigue," Angel Longevity Medical Center, https://www.angellongevity.com/blog/how-modern-lifestyles-are-leading-to-adrenal-fatigue-syndrome/.

29. Kathryn R. Simpson, *Overcoming Adrenal Fatigue: How to Restore Hormonal Balance and Feel Renewed, Energized, and Stress Free* (Oakland, CA: New Harbinger, 2011), 38.
30. Andreas Yiallouris et al., "Adrenal Aging and Its Implications on Stress Responsiveness in Humans," *Frontiers in Endocrinology* 10 (February 7, 2019): 54, https://doi.org/10.3389/fendo.2019.00054.
31. Ariana M Chao et al., "Stress, Cortisol, and Other Appetite-Related Hormones: Prospective Prediction of 6-Month Changes in Food Cravings and Weight," *Obesity (Silver Spring, MD)* 25, no. 4 (2017): 713–20, https://doi.org/10.1002/oby.21790; Centers for Disease Control and Prevention, "Insulin Resistance and Diabetes," last reviewed June 20, 2022, https://www.cdc.gov/diabetes/basics/insulin-resistance.html.
32. Simpson, *Overcoming Adrenal Fatigue*, 31.
33. James L. Wilson, *Adrenal Fatigue: The 21st Century Stress Syndrome* (Petaluma, CA: Smart Publications, 2001), 126, 134–35, 194–200.
34. Simpson, *Overcoming Adrenal Fatigue*, 83.
35. Cleveland Clinic, "Hypothyroidism," last reviewed April 19, 2020, https://my.clevelandclinic.org/health/diseases/12120-hypothyroidism.
36. Cleveland Clinic, "Hypothyroidism."
37. Simpson, *Overcoming Adrenal Fatigue*, 83.
38. "Hashimoto's Disease," MedlinePlus - Health Information from the National Library of Medicine, accessed October 5, 2023, https://medlineplus.gov/genetics/condition/hashimotos-disease/#frequency.
39. Savannah Young, "Everything You Need to Know About Hashimoto's Disease," Prime Health, July 10, 2023, https://primehealthdenver.com/hashimotos-disease/.
40. Young, "Everything You Need to Know About Hashimoto's Disease."
41. Fátima O. Martins and Silvia V. Conde, "Impact of Diet Composition on Insulin Resistance," *Nutrients* 14, no. 18 (September 9, 2022): 3716, https://doi.org/10.3390/nu14183716.
42. Centers for Disease Control and Prevention, "Type 2 Diabetes," last reviewed April 18, 2023, https://www.cdc.gov/diabetes/basics/type2.html.
43. "National Diabetes Statistics Report," Centers for Disease Control and Prevention, 2022, https://www.cdc.gov/diabetes/data/statistics-report/index.html.
44. Centers for Disease Control and Prevention, "Diabetes Risk Factors," last reviewed April 5, 2022, https://www.cdc.gov/diabetes/basics/risk-factors.html.
45. "Insulin Resistance & Prediabetes," National Institute of Diabetes and Digestive and Kidney Diseases, last modified May 22, 2018, https://www.niddk.nih.gov/health-information/diabetes/overview/what-is-diabetes

/prediabetes-insulin-resistance#:~:text=the%20normal%20range.-,What%20is%20insulin%20resistance%3F,help%20glucose%20enter%20your%20cells.
46. Centers for Disease Control and Prevention, "The Surprising Truth About Prediabetes," last reviewed July 7, 2022, https://www.cdc.gov/diabetes/library/features/truth-about-prediabetes.html.
47. Centers for Disease Control and Prevention, "Diabetes Symptoms," last reviewed September 7, 2023, https://www.cdc.gov/diabetes/basics/symptoms.html.
48. National Institute of Diabetes and Digestive and Kidney Diseases, "Type 2 Diabetes," last reviewed May 2017, https://www.niddk.nih.gov/health-information/diabetes/overview/what-is-diabetes/type-2-diabetes.
49. National Institute of Diabetes and Digestive and Kidney Diseases, "Insulin Resistance & Prediabetes," last reviewed May 22, 2018, https://www.niddk.nih.gov/health-information/diabetes/overview/what-is-diabetes/prediabetes-insulin-resistance.
50. Centers for Disease Control and Prevention, "National Diabetes Statistics Report," last reviewed November 29, 2023, https://www.cdc.gov/diabetes/data/statistics-report/coexisting-conditions-complications.html.

7. Overcome the Battle with Stress

1. Isa Kay, "Is Your Mood Disorder a Symptom of Unstable Blood Sugar?", School of Public Health, University of Michigan, October 21, 2019, https://sph.umich.edu/pursuit/2019posts/mood-blood-sugar-kujawski.html.
2. Villanova University, "Stress Management," https://www1.villanova.edu/university/health-services/health-wellness-resources/stress-management-tips.html.
3. GI Society, "Ulcer Disease," Canadian Society of Intestinal Research, https://badgut.org/information-centre/a-z-digestive-topics/ulcer-disease/.
4. Cleveland Clinic, "Parasympathetic Nervous System (PSNS)," last reviewed June 6, 2022, https://my.clevelandclinic.org/health/body/23266-parasympathetic-nervous-system-psns.
5. Mayo Clinic, "Chronic Stress Puts Your Health at Risk," August 1, 2023, https://www.mayoclinic.org/healthy-lifestyle/stress-management/in-depth/stress/art-20046037.
6. American Psychological Association, "Stress Effects on the Body," last updated March 8, 2023, https://www.apa.org/topics/stress/body.
7. Mayo Clinic, "Stress Symptoms: Effects on Your Body and Behavior," August 10, 2023 https://www.mayoclinic.org/healthy-lifestyle/stress-management/in-depth/stress-symptoms/art-20050987.
8. Mayo Clinic, "Stress Symptoms."

9. American Psychological Association, "Stress Effects on the Body."
10. Dr. Henry Cloud and Dr. John Townsend, *Boundaries: When to Say Yes, How to Say No to Take Control of Your Life* (Grand Rapids, MI: Zondervan, 1992).
11. American Psychological Association, "Stress Effects on the Body."
12. Mayo Clinic, "Post-Traumatic Stress Disorder (PTSD)," December 13, 2022, https://www.mayoclinic.org/diseases-conditions/post-traumatic-stress-disorder/symptoms-causes/syc-20355967.
13. Dimosthenis Vasiloudis, "The Enigmatic Pashupati Seal: The First Depiction of Yoga?", The Archaeologist, December 27, 2023, https://www.thearchaeologist.org/blog/category/Indus+Valley.
14. Alex Shashkevich, "Stanford Scholar Discusses Buddhism and Its Origins," Stanford News, August 20, 2018, https://news.stanford.edu/2018/08/20/stanford-scholar-discusses-buddhism-origins/.
15. Vasiloudis, "Enigmatic Pashupati Seal."
16. National Center for Complementary and Integrative Health, "Yoga: What You Need to Know," last updated August 2023, https://www.nccih.nih.gov/health/yoga-what-you-need-to-know.
17. Rebecca E. Williams and Pamela Crane, "How to Use Yoga for Emotional Well-Being," Psyche, June 7, 2023, https://psyche.co/guides/how-to-use-yoga-to-improve-your-emotional-wellbeing.
18. National Center for Complementary and Integrative Health, "Yoga: What You Need to Know."
19. Grant Hilary Brenner, "13 Real Benefits of Yoga," *Psychology Today*, September 17, 2021, https://www.psychologytoday.com/us/blog/psychiatry-the-people/202109/13-real-benefits-yoga.
20. Cari Jo Clark et al., "Trauma-Sensitive Yoga as an Adjunct Mental Health Treatment in Group Therapy for Survivors of Domestic Violence: A Feasibility Study," *Complementary Therapies in Clinical Practice* 20, no. 3 (2014): 152–58, https://doi.org/10.1016/j.ctcp.2014.04.003.
21. Mayo Clinic, "Meditation: A Simple, Fast Way to Reduce Stress," December 14, 2023, https://www.mayoclinic.org/tests-procedures/meditation/in-depth/meditation/art-20045858.
22. Julia C. Basso et al., "Brief, daily meditation enhances attention, memory, mood, and emotional regulation in non-experienced meditators," *Behavioural Brain Research* 356 (2019), 208–20.
23. Cleveland Clinic, "5 Yoga Poses You Can Do Right Now to Strengthen Your Core," June 26, 2023, https://health.clevelandclinic.org/yoga-poses-that-can-strengthen-your-core-muscles.
24. Brenner, "13 Real Benefits of Yoga."

25. Andrew Porterfield, "Study Finds a Lack of Adequate Hydration Among the Elderly," UCLA Newsroom, March 5, 2019, https://newsroom.ucla.edu/releases/study-finds-a-lack-of-adequate-hydration-among-the-elderly.
26. Tanjaniina Laukkanen et al., "Recovery from Sauna Bathing Favorably Modulates Cardiac Autonomic Nervous System," *Complementary Therapies in Medicine* 45 (2019): 190–97, https://doi.org/10.1016/j.ctim.2019.06.011.

8. Maintain a Positive Emotional Life

1. Nuraly S. Akimbekov and Mohammed S. Razzaque, "Laughter Therapy: A Humor-Induced Hormonal Intervention to Reduce Stress and Anxiety," *Current Research in Physiology* 4 (2021): 135–38, https://doi.org/10.1016/j.crphys.2021.04.002.
2. Madhuleena Roy Chowdhury, "The Neuroscience of Gratitude and Effects on the Brain," Positive Psychology, April 9, 2019, https://positivepsychology.com/neuroscience-of-gratitude/.
3. Yasuhiro Kotera, Miles Richardson, and David Sheffield, "Effects of Shinrin-Yoku (Forest Bathing) and Nature Therapy on Mental Health: A Systematic Review and Meta-analysis," *International Journal of Mental Health and Addiction* 20, no. 1 (2020): 337–61.
4. Kotera et al., "Effects of Shinrin-Yoku."
5. Moffitt Cancer Center, "Color Your World to Relieve Stress," November 16, 2018, https://endeavor.moffitt.org/archive/color-your-world-to-relieve-stress/.
6. "Can Thoughts Influence the Expression of Genes? Science Says Yes, Under Certain Conditions," Forbes, September 20, 2017, https://www.forbes.com/sites/quora/2017/09/20/can-thoughts-influence-the-expression-of-genes-science-says-yes-under-certain-conditions/?sh=4f909e47eab2.

9. Guard Your Mental Health

1. Marie Kondo, *The Life-Changing Magic of Tidying Up: The Japanese Art of Decluttering and Organizing* (Berkeley: Ten Speed, 2014).
2. Donna H. Ryan and Sarah Ryan Yockey, "Weight Loss and Improvement in Comorbidity: Differences at 5%, 10%, 15%, and Over," *Current Obesity Reports* 6, no. 2 (2017): 187–94, https://doi.org/10.1007/s13679-017-0262-y.
3. Centers for Disease Control and Prevention, "Depression Is Not a Normal Part of Growing Older," last reviewed September 14, 2022, https://www.cdc.gov/aging/depression/index.html.
4. Centers for Disease Control and Prevention, "Depression Is Not a Normal Part of Growing Older."

5. Centers for Disease Control and Prevention, "Depression Is Not a Normal Part of Growing Older."
6. Mayo Clinic, "Natural Remedies for Depression: Are They Effective?", last modified September 11, 2018, https://www.mayoclinic.org/diseases-conditions/depression/expert-answers/natural-remedies-for-depression/faq-20058026.
7. American Association for Geriatric Psychiatry, "Anxiety and Older Adults: Overcoming Worry and Fear," October 27, 2022, https://www.aagponline.org/patient-article/anxiety-and-older-adults-overcoming-worry-and-fear/.
8. Sian Ferguson, "Is Anxiety Genetic?", Healthline, June 27, 2019, https://www.healthline.com/health/mental-health/is-anxiety-genetic.
9. World Health Organization, "Anxiety Disorders," September 27, 2023, https://www.who.int/news-room/fact-sheets/detail/anxiety-disorders.
10. Ferguson, "Is Anxiety Genetic?"
11. Debra Manzella, "Reactive Hypoglycemia Overview," Verywell Health, October 24, 2023, https://www.verywellhealth.com/what-to-know-about-reactive-hypoglycemia-1087744.
12. Harvard T. H. Chan School of Public Health, "Carbohydrates and Blood Sugar," https://www.hsph.harvard.edu/nutritionsource/carbohydrates/carbohydrates-and-blood-sugar/; Linda Rath, "The Link Between Low Blood Sugar and Anxiety," WebMD, May 24, 2022, https://www.webmd.com/diabetes/low-blood-sugar-anxiety-link.
13. Manzella, "Reactive Hypoglycemia Overview."
14. Brent A. Bauer, "Is There an Effective Herbal Treatment for Anxiety?", Mayo Clinic, March 2, 2018, https://www.mayoclinic.org/diseases-conditions/generalized-anxiety-disorder/expert-answers/herbal-treatment-for-anxiety/faq-20057945; WebMD, "Natural Remedies to Alleviate Anxiety," medically reviewed by Smitha Bhandari, December 10, 2022, https://www.webmd.com/anxiety-panic/natural-remedies-for-anxiety; Crystal Raypole, "Marijuana and Anxiety: It's Complicated," medically reviewed by Alan Carter, December 16, 2019, https://www.healthline.com/health/marijuana-and-anxiety.
15. Cleveland Clinic, "Is It Normal to Get Depressed or Anxious as You Age?", December 19, 2019, https://health.clevelandclinic.org/not-normal-mental-health-problems-age.

10. Created for Work, Community, and Balance

1. "Historical Background and Development of Social Security," Social Security Administration, https://www.ssa.gov/history/briefhistory3.html.

Notes

2. National Institute on Aging, "Loneliness and Social Isolation—Tips for Staying Connected," last reviewed January 14, 2021, https://www.nia.nih.gov/health/loneliness-and-social-isolation/loneliness-and-social-isolation-tips-staying-connected.
3. Kenji Matsushita et al., "Periodontal Disease and Periodontal Disease-Related Bacteria Involved in the Pathogenesis of Alzheimer's Disease," *Journal of Inflammation Research* 13 (June 30, 2020): 275–83, https://doi.org/10.2147/JIR.S255309.
4. Gaétan Chevalier et al., "Earthing: Health Implications of Reconnecting the Human Body to the Earth's Surface Electrons," *Journal of Environmental and Public Health* 2012 (2012): 291541, https://doi.org/10.1155/2012/291541.
5. Ryan Raman, "What Does Magnesium Do for Your Body?", Healthline, July 14, 2023, https://www.healthline.com/nutrition/what-does-magnesium-do.

12. Healthy Habits for a Long Life

1. Crystal Raypole, "6 Ways to Rewire Your Brain," Healthline, medically reviewed by Timothy J. Legg, PhD, PsyD, June 17, 2020, https://www.healthline.com/health/rewiring-your-brain.
2. Caroline Leaf, *Think and Eat Yourself Smart: A Neuroscientific Approach to a Sharper Mind and Healthier Life* (Ada, MI: Baker Books, 2016), 101–2.

Appendix: Fall Prevention

1. Centers for Disease Control and Prevention, "Keep on Your Feet," last modified March 24, 2023, https://www.cdc.gov/injury/features/older-adult-falls/index.html.
2. Mayo Clinic, "Fall Prevention: Simple Tips to Prevent Falls," February 3, 2022, https://www.mayoclinic.org/healthy-lifestyle/healthy-aging/in-depth/fall-prevention/art-20047358.

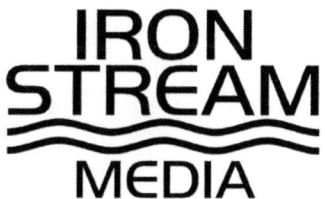

If you enjoyed this book, will you consider sharing the message with others?

Let us know your thoughts. You can let the author know by visiting or sharing a photo of the cover on our social media pages or leaving a review at a retailer's site. All of it helps us get the message out!

Email: info@ironstreammedia.com

   @ironstreammedia

Iron Stream, Iron Stream Fiction, Iron Stream Kids, Brookstone Publishing Group, and Life Bible Study are imprints of Iron Stream Media, which derives its name from Proverbs 27:17, "As iron sharpens iron, so one person sharpens another." This sharpening describes the process of discipleship, one to another. With this in mind, Iron Stream Media provides a variety of solutions for churches, ministry leaders, and nonprofits ranging from in-depth Bible study curriculum and Christian book publishing to custom publishing and consultative services.

For more information on ISM and its imprints, please visit
IronStreamMedia.com

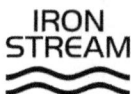 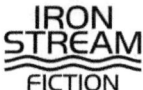 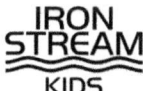

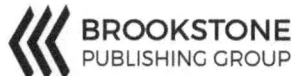